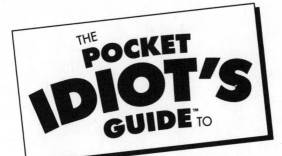

THE POCKET IDIOT'S GUIDE™ TO

Great Abs

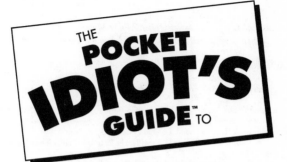

Great Abs

by Tom Seabourne, Ph.D.

ALPHA

A member of the Penguin Group (USA) Inc.

This book is dedicated to Jeff Tuller, Mindy Mylrea, and the thousands of fitness professionals around the world trying to make a difference.

ALPHA BOOKS

Published by the Penguin Group

Penguin Group (USA) Inc., 375 Hudson Street, New York, New York 10014, U.S.A.

Penguin Group (Canada), 10 Alcorn Avenue, Toronto, Ontario, Canada M4V 3B2 (a division of Pearson Penguin Canada Inc.)

Penguin Books Ltd, 80 Strand, London WC2R 0RL, England

Penguin Ireland, 25 St Stephen's Green, Dublin 2, Ireland (a division of Penguin Books Ltd)

Penguin Group (Australia), 250 Camberwell Road, Camberwell, Victoria 3124, Australia (a division of Pearson Australia Group Pty Ltd)

Penguin Books India Pvt Ltd, 11 Community Centre, Panchsheel Park, New Delhi—110 017, India

Penguin Group (NZ), cnr Airborne and Rosedale Roads, Albany, Auckland 1310, New Zealand (a division of Pearson New Zealand Ltd)

Penguin Books (South Africa) (Pty) Ltd, 24 Sturdee Avenue, Rosebank, Johannesburg 2196, South Africa

Penguin Books Ltd, Registered Offices: 80 Strand, London WC2R 0RL, England

International Standard Book Number: 1-59257-441-6
Library of Congress Catalog Card Number: 2005932768

07   06   8   7   6   5   4   3   2

Interpretation of the printing code: The rightmost number of the first series of numbers is the year of the book's printing; the rightmost number of the second series of numbers is the number of the book's printing. For example, a printing code of 05-1 shows that the first printing occurred in 2005.

Printed in the United States of America

Note: This publication contains the opinions and ideas of its author. It is intended to provide helpful and informative material on the subject matter covered. It is sold with the understanding that the author and publisher are not engaged in rendering professional services in the book. If the reader requires personal assistance or advice, a competent professional should be consulted.

The author and publisher specifically disclaim any responsibility for any liability, loss, or risk, personal or otherwise, which is incurred as a consequence, directly or indirectly, of the use and application of any of the contents of this book.

Most Alpha books are available at special quantity discounts for bulk purchases for sales promotions, premiums, fund-raising, or educational use. Special books, or book excerpts, can also be created to fit specific needs.

For details, write: Special Markets, Alpha Books, 375 Hudson Street, New York, NY 10014.

Contents

Introduction

You probably have done stomach exercises until you are blue in the face. Why isn't your waistline in the kind of shape it should be? How would you like to have great abs without doing hundreds of sit-ups or crunches? This is an incredible program that combines all of the components you need to have flat abs—and it's not as difficult as you may think.

Change the way you move and think. We take normal activities in and out of the gym and transform them into flab-burning fun. Photos and illustrations will provide you with perfect patterns to follow. At the same time, you will learn exactly what to eat to fuel your muscles and starve your fat cells.

Start a mind-body journey to lose your gut. Unlike other books, our program weaves together a sensible eating plan, do-able activities, and the mental strategies you will need to reach your ab-solute genetic potential. We start you off easy, and then as you get leaner and stronger, you can keep your abs-sculpting workout challenging and productive.

Men want their abs rock-hard, ripped, and defined while women prefer them to be sleek, tight, and flat. Men want to lose their love-handles and women will gladly give away their pooch (the pooch is that area just below the belly button that just sort of pooches out.) You will learn specific in-the-home/office and gym exercises that will target all of your trouble spots.

Our book is chock-full of a variety of movement choices and eating strategies to provide you with a balanced approach to achieving those ideal abs. You will learn how to use a variety of eating styles, which include six, five, four, or even just three meals a day to reach your goals.

Imagine for a moment what it would feel like to lose an inch around your waist in a week. Think of how that would make you feel. It's not impossible. It's completely within your grasp. You can do this now. This program could be the best thing you have ever done for yourself.

Prepare for your one-stop shop to flat abs. No more painful hours on treadmills or ab-shapers. No hundreds of sets and reps and trying to stay in your fat-burning zone. Instead, great abs are yours by making small changes that lead to big results. You have seen great abs on people who never stepped foot into a gym or counted a calorie. You can be one of those people.

In This Book

Motivation. Successful people exercise and eat correctly. Even President Bush has time to work out. You feel more energetic and confident. It takes about a month to reinvent yourself. Every day your Great Abs program gets easier.

Diet. At first, you ate the meat but not the bun. That didn't work, so you ate the bun but threw out the meat. Your body gets lean when you eat foods in combination (the whole-grain bun and the meat), along with fruits and veggies.

Exercise. Train at home while watching TV or listening to music. Instead of lifelessly watching a sitcom, dance. Your body loves to move.

Isolation exercises sculpt your midsection. Do these at home, in your office, or in the gym. Train your torso while typing on your computer or during your lunch break. To chisel those abs, stimulate them.

In this book you will find sidebars that are tidbits of important and useful information to keep you making progress on the program.

 Bet You Didn't Know _____

This sidebar warns you of common myths and misconceptions concerning diet and exercise.

Get It Right _____

This sidebar provides you with cautionary warnings to be sure you're doing your exercises right.

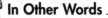

In Other Words

This sidebar helps you to understand the anatomy of your abs and figure out technical or unusual terms and concepts found in the main text. For example, rectus abdominis or quadratus lumborum.

Your Personal Trainer

This sidebar provides you with quick tips about how to do your exercises correctly and information to keep your form perfect.

Acknowledgments

I want to thank the photographer, Ron Barker, and our fabulous models, Brittany Scott and Brandon Sears. Thanks to Paul Dinas, Phil Kitchel, Emily Bell, and Billy Fields for their amazing coaching along the way. My wife, Danese, and five beautiful children Alaina, Grant, Laura, Susanna, and Julia are always finding new ways to make workouts fun. And finally to my brother, Rick, my sister, Barb, and my mother, Ann, who, in my opinion, own the finest fitness facility in northeastern Pennsylvania.

Special Thanks to the Technical Reviewer

The Pocket Idiot's Guide to Great Abs was reviewed by an expert who double-checked the accuracy of what you'll learn here, to help us ensure that this book gives you everything you need to know. Special thanks are extended to Shannon Loveless.

Trademarks

All terms mentioned in this book that are known to be or are suspected of being trademarks or service marks have been appropriately capitalized. Alpha Books and Penguin Group (USA) Inc. cannot attest to the accuracy of this information. Use of a term in this book should not be regarded as affecting the validity of any trademark or service mark.

Chapter 1

Body Made Simple

In This Chapter

- Trimming tools to sculpt your abs
- Your abs—a powerful combination
- The "secret" ab muscle
- Navel maneuvers to beat the pooch
- Washboard wisdom—PE 101

The one muscle group that never goes out of style is your abdominals. Advertisers have hooked people into thinking that a tight midsection is the ultimate goal. Your waistline is treated differently than your back or legs. Men size up other men by a quick glance at the size of their belly. Popular magazines exhort women to banish their midriffs by strapping on belly-tightening girdles. Straight skirts are worn to conceal the embarrassing bulges and pooch.

It is important to begin with the anatomy and function of your abs so that you will better understand the training concepts that will be presented later. Most people don't seem to notice that the abs are connected to the rest of the body. By understanding how each abdominal muscle functions, you'll be able to work your abs efficiently, to firm and tone them to their full potential. If you understand the location and function of each ab muscle, you will get a good feel of how they actually work. There are four major muscle groups in the abdominal region, and a couple of other eye-catching muscles in the surrounding area. Contrary to general thought, your abs aren't just in the front of your stomach. They are an amazing pattern of muscles connected to your hips, ribcage, and your backbone. To have great abs, you need to do belly exercises, lower-back moves, and side-of-your-stomach toners.

 Your Personal Trainer _____

Sit and stand with perfect posture and your lower pooch will all but disappear.

Your abs include four muscle groups:

1. Your six-pack or rectus abdominis
2. Your side abs or external obliques
3. Your internal obliques, underneath your side abs
4. Underneath all of these muscles, your transverse abdominis

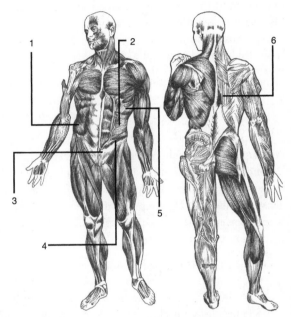

1. External Oblique
2. Internal Oblique
3. Rectus abdominus

4. Transverse abdominus
5. Serratis anterior
6. Erector Spinae

The muscle groups in your abdomen.

Rectus Abdominis

Your rectus abdominis is a wide, flat sheath of muscle, commonly referred to as your six-pack. It stretches from the bottom of the ribs down to just below the navel (belly button). The six-pack is not six muscles. It is visible sections of a single muscle. It is similar to your thigh muscle, but with partitions. The partitions are fibrous bands called tendinous inscriptions.

When you flex your rectus abdominis muscle to lean forward, your lower back bends about 30 degrees. The rectus abdominis is responsible for bending forward at the waist and drawing your pelvis upward.

These front stomach muscles pull your chest toward your hips. In essence, the main thing your front stomach muscles do is decrease the distance between your chest and hips.

Great care and excellent technique are required to strengthen the abdominal muscles. To be effective, you must pull your chest toward the knees using only the abdominal group. Often, however, other, more powerful muscles (those that flex the legs and hips) do much of the work.

Sounds like toning your stomach is a job for the good old sit-up you did in P.E. class. The problem with regular sit-ups is that you work every other muscle besides your abs. You pull on your neck, and your legs do most of the work because you have someone holding your ankles. Traditional sit-ups emphasize sitting up rather than pulling your chest toward your hips. Most people tend to compromise their form when reaching their fatigue level, and a common mistake people make is pulling on their neck when tired.

Sit-ups are inefficient because the hip flexor works best when the legs are straight as they are when doing sit-ups. The hip flexor muscle lies underneath your abs and connects the lower part of your spine to your upper leg. Its main function is to raise your leg in front of you. When you flex it, your leg raises. If you anchor your ankles for a sit-up, your hip flexor does most of the work in pulling your chest toward your knees. Worse than that, regular sit-ups grind the vertebrae in your lower back.

Get It Right

To maintain your eye-catching abs, take the hip flexors out of your ab exercises.

Exercises presented in the home, office, and gym sections of this book show you ways to take the hip flexors out of the equation.

Just as you can't contract half of your thigh, you can't contract half of your abs. There goes the notion of training your "upper abs" and "lower abs" in complete isolation. However, you can focus on the upper bundles of muscle fiber by moving just the torso or the lower fibers by moving the hips.

If you have well-defined upper abs and you can't see your lower abs, it's not that your lower abs need more work. It just means you've got fat covering them. Read Chapters 8 and 9 to learn how to shed the fat to exhibit those lower abs.

Your upper abs are stimulated when you do crunches without resistance, but when you add resistance the lower abs work equally as much. Reverse crunches work the lower abs more than the upper abs, but the obliques also help in that exercise. The lesson here is that when you add resistance to an abdominal exercise, all of your ab muscles join in to get the job done.

You might be afraid to add resistance to your ab exercises for fear of developing muscular love handles, but since the side-ab abdominal wall is a sheet of muscle, even if you add resistance to your side-ab exercises the muscle is unlikely to protrude. Your side-ab muscles don't have the capacity to expand like your front-ab muscles do. A large waist comes from a lot of fat in that area, a large pelvic girdle, or a beer belly.

Side Abs

A safe guess is that you want to cut and define your conductor muscle (your six-pack), but what about the orchestra (your side abs)? The conductor is only as good as the orchestra, and your six-pack would be better looking if you spent time developing the side abs as well.

Love handles are those rolls of fat that you can pinch on the sides of your waist. Your well-defined six-pack is adulterated by a matching set of love handles. But just beneath this layer of fluff is a power set of muscles called your obliques.

Although you cannot spot reduce your love handles, you can tone the oblique muscles underneath. Do this and your waistline will be firmer, flatter, and tighter. And when you shed the fat that surrounds them, your entire waistline will be cut and defined.

Tone your obliques while whittling away your love handles. Love handles generally disappear in men when their percentage of body fat drops into the single digits. Women only have to get their body fat level down to about 15 percent.

External Obliques

Your external obliques are the muscles at the sides of the waist—the sexy muscles under your love handles. They form a "V" shape from the ribs down to below your navel. Tuck your fingers into your front pockets. That is the shape of your external obliques.

Your external obliques are used when you twist and bend forward. They are activated by twisting in your chair, or bending down to pick up that pen on the floor. Strong obliques help to pull, lift, or push heavy objects. Your obliques are the only abdominal muscles constantly active during standing. They function while you are in an upright posture to brace your torso. Together, these muscles contract to tilt the torso, as well as twist it, from side to side. They steady your torso to keep gravity from pulling you out of balance.

Your external obliques help with your crunches and they brace your spine. Your oblique muscles are interwoven all the way around your middle. This provides lower-back support when you move. If the waist moves, the external obliques are involved. The torso rotation in golf and tennis is mostly done by the external obliques.

Even the basic crunch motion wouldn't be possible without a strong, flexed set of external obliques to steady your torso. Well-developed obliques make your waist tighter. The external obliques are the largest of the abdominal muscles.

Internal Obliques

Your internal obliques are underneath your external obliques. They extend diagonally down the sides of your waist forming an inverted "V" from your pelvis to your lower ribs. Your internal obliques run in the opposite direction as your external obliques.

Your obliques are thin muscles. They are not designed for heavy resistance training. They enclose your organs. Similar to the externals, the internal obliques are involved in torso rotation. You also use these muscles when you breathe deeply. Both the internal and external obliques are responsible for the twisting movement of your torso and side bends. For your torso to twist, your internal oblique and the opposite external oblique flex. If you wanted to bend to one side, both the internal and external obliques on the same side flex simultaneously. That is why "oblique twists" work well to train these muscles. When you do these exercises, curl your trunk forward and diagonally so that your left armpit moves toward your right hip.

A great toning exercise for these muscles is the side plank. Another exercise that uses the rotating capabilities of your internal obliques is the "scissors." Your obliques are used in almost every move you make, so train them well.

Although your obliques are not designed to grow huge no matter how hard you train them, keep them strong to maintain ideal postural alignment.

If you happen to be one of the unfortunate genetically gifted few whose sides grow larger from oblique work, then minimize your oblique training.

Transverse Abdominis

The transverse abdominis (TVA) muscle lies beneath all of your other abdominal muscles, and therefore cannot be felt with your hands nor can it be seen. It's a thin muscle that runs horizontally, surrounding your abdomen.

Although this muscle is invisible, your TVA is responsible for keeping your waist nicely tucked in. When you suck in your stomach to look skinny you are using your TVA. You can feel it flex when you cough or sneeze. Think of it as a girdle because it functions as a compressor for the abdomen, keeping everything in place. It contracts when the other ab muscles are working. The TVA does not bend your spine. It serves as a brace for your lower back.

 Bet You Didn't Know

> The *kiai* in karate trains your TVA. So does the forceful breathing of Lamaze.

Training your TVA is easy. From the beginning position of any ab exercise, exhale slowly and use your abs to gently draw in the sides of your torso as you bring your lower ribs toward your hips. Bring your navel as close as possible to your spine.

Imagine you're wearing a girdle or weight-lifting belt. Pull it tight. Now tighten it another notch. This is your TVA in action, creating the appearance of a smaller waist. Train this muscle daily, and your TVA (and obliques) will be the only weight-lifting belt that you will ever need. But activating your TVA takes concentration and practice.

The Intercostals

The intercostals are the breathing muscles that lie between your ribs. They are bands of muscle angling downward in the sides of the rib cage and the upper abdomen. The intercostals flex the torso and cause it to twist, so doing any type of elbow-to-opposite-knee exercise will stimulate this group of muscles.

The Serratus

The serratus anterior muscles are the fingerlike strands of muscle on the rib cage between the front abs and the lats. You can feel them flex when you attempt to lower your ribcage.

Your serratus muscles make your upper body look more defined when you have little *subcutaneous fat*. The serratus helps when you push heavy objects off your chest at various angles, controls the separation of your shoulder blades, and assists in lifting your shoulders. If you're very lean and muscular, your serratus and external obliques form a criss-cross of muscular definition. The "fingers to toes" exercise trains your serratus.

In Other Words

Subcutaneous fat is the adipose tissue between your skin and ab muscles that smoothes out definition.

Back muscles co-contract with your ab muscles to perform the exercises in this program. The back muscles are called the *erector spinae*, and they run the entire length of your spine on either side of your vertebrae. They bend your spine backward and sideways and act as a brace.

Your back muscles also counterbalance your movement when your abs flex and you lean forward. No abs program is complete without training your back: strong abs equal a strong back, and vice versa. If you ignore your back while strengthening your abdominals, you encourage and promote poor posture.

That's why this book has several exercises that train your abs and back simultaneously. Our other *Pocket Idiot's Guides* also have other exercises such as squats, dead lifts, and the bench press that, when performed with enough intensity, tax the abs as stabilizers better than almost anything else.

Strong pelvic floor muscles are crucial to a strong back. When you contract the pelvic floor muscles (by doing a kegal exercise) at the same time as you contract your transverse abdominis, other deep muscles in your back are activated. These muscles are directly responsible for bracing your spine during your ab training.

Firm, tight abs make you look and feel better. Every time you move, your abs are involved. In the following chapters, you will learn exercises that you can perform at home, at work, or while waiting in line. Don't wait. You can begin your training right now while reading this paragraph. Simply exhale and contract your abs by bringing your lower back flat into your chair. Read the rest of this book and you can get the abs you've always dreamed of.

Brain Training: Do It, but Do It Right

In This Chapter

- Change your life
- With a partner or on your own
- Extra inches won't control you
- Better results with less effort

You are an athlete! Even though you may not look the part, and even if your strong, powerful midsection is hidden under a layer of fat, you're an athlete, so treat yourself like one. An athlete warms up, works out, cools down, and stretches.

Set your goal—flat sculpted abs, or just being able to button your pants—and prepare to totally focus. Quick goals keep you pumped up for the long haul, so set a goal such as losing a couple of inches around your waist in two weeks. Don't compare your progress to others. It's your workout, not theirs.

You may prefer to train your abs at home, in the office, in a gym, or all of the above. Your personality may dictate a strict regimen, or you may never do the same exercise twice in a row.

 Your Personal Trainer

> Get pumped up by listening to your favorite music. Imagine yourself lean and ripped and focusing on your ultimate goal.

Brain Training Is Key

Make a choice. You may decide that it is easier to be flabby than to work out and eat right. If you choose to be overweight, be aware that your choice means it's harder to walk up a flight of stairs and you have to buy new clothes every six months.

But if you choose to work out, be very specific about your goals. Concrete goals keep you on the program long enough to see results. Before you begin working out, imagine how you will feel after a few months of training. Your clothes will fit better, you will feel better, and you will look better. Whenever you don't feel like tying your shoes, think about where you will be after six months of activity. Once you see results, you will be hooked. Change your mind about your body. Make a commitment to be positive so that you will be one of the few, the proud, the fit. Photos in fitness magazines, fitness programs on TV, and the photos in this book will keep you inspired. While you are reading this book, press your lower back into the chair. Look at your abs. They're working! Just by flexing your abs a couple of times an hour your muscle tone will improve and your pooch will disappear.

You've probably tried other programs and quit. Remember this: *You didn't fail, the program failed.* Relax. Once you stop obsessing about flat abs they will be easier to attain. Stress increases the hormone cortisol, leading to an increase in belly fat.

Don't try to do too much too soon. Magazines and infomercials try to coerce you into working out at a certain pace or using certain form. Look past the "buy today" ad and you will see that there is no quick fix to sleek, sexy abs. Instant results don't happen. It is better to lose an inch a week than to lose three inches a week and gain six inches back in a month. You are looking for progress, not perfection.

Most successful people write their goals and keep track of their progress. That is certainly not a requirement for this program, but keeping a log of your workouts can increase your motivation. Writing down how long you walked or how much weight you lifted is proof positive that you are making progress.

Anything Can Be Your Thing

You don't have to jog or run to lose your belly. There are no hard and fast rules for losing fat around your waist. There are ab devices and aerobicizer machines, but your midsection doesn't know whether you are using an expensive piece of equipment or not. Your muscles firm up when they are challenged.

Try new activities to keep your workouts progressing. Any exercise that you love will work. Be creative about getting off the couch. Dance around the living room or take your dog for a walk—even if you don't have one.

Your body adapts to whatever you do. If you sit around all of the time, your body expects you to be sedentary. Start moving and your body will come alive. You were meant to move, not sit at a desk or in your car all day.

Start your program and progress gradually. Teach your body how much more fun it is to move than it is to be still. Exercise reduces the symptoms of depression and makes you feel better about yourself. Your circulation increases and you are more creative.

To be conscientious and productive, turn work into play. Go for a bike ride, in-line skate, or hit a tennis ball against a wall. If you prefer working out with people, play volleyball or softball. If you love to run or swim but don't want to do it because you are not efficient, do it anyway. You burn more fat when you are not efficient. All those extra calories you use while you are splaying your elbows or splashing around slice away the fat surrounding your beautiful abs.

A balanced program works. Start with baby steps. If it doesn't feel good, don't do it. You are a creature of habit. Set up habits that keep you on your program.

Integrating Workouts and Life

Some people love the feeling of working out. If that is you, then you will stick to the program. Training will be an end in itself. But if you hate every second of your activity you must find a way to make it worthwhile. Listen to books on tape, watch the news, or contemplate the universe. Do whatever it takes to keep moving. Look forward to your workout or you won't do it. You find a way to do the things that you enjoy. If you don't want to do something, you find a way to quit. Excuses include lack of time, injury, negative emotions, poor social support, or low motivation.

When you begin your program with your home, office, or gym workouts, make them effortless. Week by week add intensity. Add enough effort to make progress. As you get fitter, your body will enjoy the challenge of greater effort.

The best time to work out is whenever fits your schedule. Once you make your abs program part of your life, it is easy. If it's in your schedule, you will do it. Working out in the morning wakes you up. It replaces coffee as a pick-me-up and turns your metabolism into a fat-burning furnace. Afternoon and evening workouts are iffy. Happy-hour dates and important appointments such as your favorite sitcom can often pre-empt your workout. But if you must work out in the evening, be sure to get done before your eyelids get heavy. Schedule your workout for a specific time and people will learn not to bother you. They will understand how important your health is.

Your whole life may change if you join a gym. Not only are gyms social clubs, but they are great places to meet workout partners. If you find a workout partner, schedule a time to meet. It's fun to have a spotter and to enjoy good conversation between sets. But be prepared if your workout partner doesn't show up. Always have a back-up workout planned. Making a trip to the gym also means you have made a commitment to work out, and you are less likely to get sidetracked as you would if you were at home or at the office.

You don't have to spend hours in a gym to get great abs, but the magic 20-minute fat-burning workout is not magic either. Split your workout into mini-workouts throughout the day for great results.

Pushing Through the Burn

Life gets in the way and that's okay. You will miss workouts occasionally. Make them up with office exercises or do something when you arrive home. If you have to leave town, stash an exercise band in your suitcase as a reminder to work out on the road. If you are a compulsive type A personality, skip a workout on purpose. The next day get right back on the wagon. This is a quick lesson teaching you that falling off the wagon is no big deal.

The first month is the worst month. Once you make your eating and exercising a habit, it's easy. Try not to miss any meals or workouts for your first month. Clear your schedule to be sure of no conflicts. Keep telling yourself that you can quit after a month. But if you do make it, and you will, reward yourself with clothing that is a couple of sizes smaller.

You will not have your best workout every day you train. Some workouts will be better than others depending on how you eat, sleep, and what type of stress you are dealing with. If you tie your shoes and don't feel like doing anything, warm up. After the warm-up decide if you can at least start your workout. Most of the time, once you start you will be fine. After your wheels are turning, momentum keeps you going.

Whatever you do, don't quit completely. Starting over is harder than cutting back. Do anything, even if it is just a walk around the block. It is so much easier to increase your intensity than it is to start from scratch.

Getting sore is not part of the program. Some people think that if they didn't get sore, the workout didn't do any good. That is simply not true. Your goal is to work out for the long haul. Soreness is not an option.

You may experience sprains, strains, aches, and pains. See your physician and ask if there is a way to work out around the problem. If you have a good medical team, they will explain to you the importance of exercise and help you to figure out a way to keep training.

Get It Right

Close your eyes and imagine your ab muscles flexing and shortening like slow-moving cables through a pulley that draws your chest and shoulders off the floor.

Before you begin your crunches, follow a ritual. Have a specific pattern to get you started with your training and you will be more likely to continue your training the day after, and the day after that. Adjust your back on the floor, keep your neck relaxed, bring your arms into position, and exhale during each repetition.

Don't rush. If you do an ab exercise incorrectly, you end up using many other muscle groups instead of your abs. You strain your neck and your back and your abs don't get a workout.

Use this technique to slow down and tune into your muscles: Lie down on your back and flex your abs by pressing your lower back into the floor for three seconds, relax. Feel the difference between the tension and relaxation in your ab muscles. Continue this exercise cycle for ten reps until you are sure you feel your abs doing the work.

This exercise teaches you to be aware of your ab muscles while you are training them. Then when you are doing your ab-isolation exercises, you will notice if you are inadvertently using other muscles.

Although you don't have to do yoga, tai chi, or pilates to get great abs, the mind-body benefits of these activities is helpful. Take a look at some of the videos in the appendix to see if you are interested in these alternative forms of ab training.

 Bet You Didn't Know

> Rehearse your ab workout in your head and it actually will send electrical signals to your ab muscles.

Keeping Your Diet On-Track

Eating rituals are important, too. Know what you are going to eat the next day. Schedule meals in advance and sit down to all of your meals. Be sure to eat enough healthy snacks so you are not ravenous. Don't obsess about food. Eat enough to fuel your muscles and be done with it. Don't let stress creep into mealtime. Eat slowly and pay attention to what you are eating.

A forbidden-food day once a week, and a week off from exercise every six months, is required. You have to stick to your plan, but you don't want to burn yourself out either. Some people become so addicted to their eating and workout program that, when they miss a day, they give up completely and succumb to what psychologists term "abstinence violation." Remember to enjoy life as well, or you won't reap the benefits of the healthier you.

Visualization

Fitness models and bodybuilders use their minds to affect their bodies. They imagine muscle fibers splitting during a workout. Then they visualize blood rushing to the muscles to nourish and rebuild them.

Visualization is effective if you get a clear mental picture of the outcome (flat abs), and the strategy you will use to get there (your workout). As an experiment, take a few minutes a day to see your "ideal abs" and mentally rehearse the workout that will get you there. Watch a mental movie of yourself working your abs. Seeing your workout before it happens is a tool. It makes your ab workout easier and more effective. If you have rehearsed your workout in your head, think how much easier it will be to do.

You can use visualization in your bed just before sleep, or while you walk, pedal, or step. When you close your eyes and imagine you are flexing your abs, there is electrical activity in your ab muscles. This is not to say that you can lie down on your bed and train in your sleep, but it is important for you to know that you can use your mind to stimulate your muscles.

In Other Words

Abstinence violation is psychobabble that means when you miss a day of your workout or eating program you decide to give up and throw in the towel.

Self Talk

You talk to yourself all of the time without knowing it. You have a choice—"I don't have time to work out today, I have yardwork" or "I can mow the lawn with a push mower for my workout."

Self-talk such as "My abs are getting ripped" gets you pumped. Always keep your self-talk positive.

Chapter 3

Ab-Solute Principles

In This Chapter

- The principles behind rock-hard abs
- Quality not quantity
- Washboard-worthy circuit
- Fast ab-toning principles
- No gut all glory—follow the plan

Training your abs works fast. A firmer stomach means you will look slimmer. You will feel better immediately and you should see visible results in as little as a few weeks. Before each workout, plan the order of your exercises and the intensity of your workout. Get psyched up for each rep.

Use the exercises that work best for you. Don't be afraid to experiment; trial and error is part of the learning process. What works the upper-stomach muscles for you might work the lower-stomach muscles for someone else.

If your abs feel like they are working, they are. Keep doing what you're doing until it doesn't work anymore. You cannot shape your ab muscles; you can make them bigger or more toned.

Form

Emphasize keeping your form perfect and maintain normal breathing. All exercises should be performed with control and in a comfortable range of motion.

Maintain perfect posture on every exercise.

Keep your stomach in; relax your neck; keep your back flat (don't arch). Don't bend too far, a few inches in either direction is all you need.

Focus on a specific part of your stomach. For example, to train the side of your stomach, concentrate on leaning forward and twisting to the side. Relax the rest of your muscles so a higher percentage of force is exerted behind the specific muscle group you are working.

Place the palm of your hand just below your navel. Pooch your stomach out as if attempting to pose for the "before" picture on an infomercial. Then use your lower-stomach muscles to slowly squeeze your lower abs toward your spine and hold for three seconds. Relax for a few seconds and try it again. Do this exercise for a few reps. Then, whenever you're performing stomach exercises, remember to flex these muscles before and during all of your reps.

Using your lower-ab muscles to pull your navel toward your spine makes all of your stomach exercises more effective. This is not the same as sucking your stomach in. It's flexing the muscles in your lower abs and pulling them toward your backbone.

Flexing these lower-stomach muscles stimulates muscles that are connected to your spine. This makes your entire stomach area more stable. More stability means that your ab muscles will produce more force and therefore tone more muscle. Flexing the lower ab muscles also keeps your back healthy.

Never let weight or repetitions dictate form.

If you are training the front of your stomach, keep your neck relaxed. The rest of your muscles should not be helping with the movement. Move smoothly into each repetition with a controlled and 100 percent energized effort.

Use the suggested range of motion on each of your ab exercises. Ease into your workout. Start with some easy repetitions, then gradually increase the intensity. Breathe normally when you are first learning the exercise. But when the exercise becomes familiar, exhale during the exertion phase of each rep. Inhale on your short rests between each contraction.

Symmetrical development of your abs and lower back is important. An unbalanced workout program decreases the flexibility in your abs and upper-thigh muscles leading to abnormal posture. Postural problems may increase the chance of injury to your under-developed back.

Fortunately this program has built-in back exercises that you perform at the same time you are training your abs.

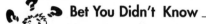

> **Bet You Didn't Know** _____
>
> Exhale on the up phase of your ab exercise. This pulls your abs inward, making sure you use the deeper muscles of your abs. Inhaling on the up phase may cause your abdomen to pooch out, causing overarching and strain to your lower back. An easy way to remember this is EE = Exhale Exertion.

Speed

Take your time on each repetition. The slower you move, the less momentum, and the more work your ab muscles are accomplishing. You should be able to stop at any point during each rep.

Three seconds in both directions works well.

During each repetition of your ab workout there are two different parts. One part is called the *positive*—the "up phase" of the repetition. The second part is the *negative* or the "down phase" of the repetition. It is important to come down slowly on the negative phase. Moving slowly on the negative phase will chisel those abs fast.

Slower uses more muscle fibers.

Some ab fans pay far too much attention to the quantity of crunches rather than to the quality of each movement. If you are too fatigued to do the negative portion of the three-second rep, maintaining absolute control of the movement, then you are done with that ab exercise for the day.

Focus on doing reps correctly, not on how many reps you should do. Your ab muscles will respond when you use good form at a controlled speed.

Cheating on your reps slows your progress and leads to possible injury, if not immediately, then down the road. Don't compare how many reps you can do to someone else's total. Compare you to you.

Resistance

There is no better way to contour and streamline your abs than using resistance. You cannot target fat around your waist, but you can tone the muscle underneath. To shrink a spreading waist, resistance training helps to speed your metabolism. Your muscle becomes toned and more compact as the surrounding fat disappears.

Use dumbbells, bands, stability balls, or weight plates to challenge your stomach muscles. Resistance bands are great for training the sides of your stomach. Stash one in your suitcase and you have your own on-the-road ab-toning device.

Your stomach muscles will tone and tighten in response to progressively increased resistance. As your stomach muscles get stronger, gradually increase the amount of weight you are using. You may also increase reps, sets, or take less rest between sets to challenge your abs.

Three important factors in your ab workouts will dictate your progress—the intensity of the stress put on the muscle, the duration of the workout, and how many times a week you train your abs.

Don't be concerned that your abs will grow huge from resistance training. Women are especially worried that they will develop huge stomach muscles and increase their waistline. Listen to your body. If your stomach muscles are stronger, more toned, and you are not gaining additional body fat, you are doing everything right.

In Other Words

The **overload principle** states that your ab muscles will continue to respond as you progressively increase the resistance.

At first, your body weight is enough resistance to train your abs. Gradually add weight. Be sure you can perform ten repetitions with perfect form before advancing to a heavier weight. As your muscles adapt, and your abs get stronger, your goal will be to do ten reps with about 75 percent of the maximum resistance that you could handle for one rep.

When you begin to use resistance for your ab training, start with a very light weight. Do not increase
your resistance more than five percent in a single
workout.

Training Strategies

If you have a busy schedule (and don't we all?), perform only one set of each exercise. In addition to
being time-efficient, single-set training is almost as
effective as multiple-set training.

Do one exercise for each ab-muscle group. Make
sure you don't duplicate movements. For example,
it makes no sense to do a set of crunches with no
resistance, and then another set of crunches with
resistance bands. Both of these exercises are exactly
the same movement and work the same specific
muscles. Instead, do a set of crunches for your over-
all midsection and then a side-ab training exercise
for the sides of your stomach.

Perform one to three sets per body part.

After you have trained for a few months, your
stomach muscles can handle more than one set of a
particular exercise. Work your way up to three sets
of ten repetitions on every ab exercise. You know
you are doing too much if you lose your form.

Losing your form means you can't finish a rep without changing your body position. If you're doing
crunches and you start bouncing off of the floor,
you're finished with the exercise. Whether you've

done one set or four sets, if you've had a break in
your form, you're done. Simply pay attention to
your form rep by rep.

Get It Right

Don't twist your elbow to your opposite knee at the top of your sit-up. This
creates torsion stress to your lower back,
and it does nothing to tone your abs.

Perform sets consecutively or in a circuit.

If one of your goals is to lose belly fat, move quickly
from one ab exercise to the next. Keep charts to
record how you are advancing in each of your muscle groups. Write down how many sets, how many
reps, how much resistance, and how much rest you
take between sets. As you increase the resistance and
the number of repetitions, your muscles will respond.

When you are ready for another challenge, do an
ab-training circuit. Perform one set of each exercise
without rest. This burns more calories than straight
sets of crunches.

Circuit training also forces your cardiovascular system to work overtime. Without resting between
sets you increase the amount of time you spend
toning those abs compared with the amount of time
you spend resting. This increases the metabolic
demand of the workout and defines those abs.

Pulse Training

Pulsing through your abdominal crunches is another way to add intensity. The principle behind pulsing is that instead of doing full crunches, you just stay at your mid-range and make a small movement up and down. Pulsing preps your abs for using more resistance because it allows you to overload the part of your ab muscles that are strongest, without being limited by the part of the movement where you're weakest.

Do 3 sets of 10 repetitions of pulsing, resting one minute between each set. Follow those with a set of 10 full range-of-motion crunches.

Reversing Sets and Reps

Choose an abdominal exercise that you have difficulty performing a single rep of. Do 10 sets of one repetition, resting 30 seconds between each set.

This is a fabulous workout because you end up performing 10 repetitions of an exercise you normally can only do 1 or 2 reps of. This program requires you to recruit more total ab-muscle fibers than usual.

Reverse your sets and reps. Take your current set and rep scheme and reverse it. Since you normally do 3 sets of 10 reps, try crunching 10 sets of 3 reps.

Since you're stopping at 3 reps instead of 10, rest 10 seconds or less between sets. Reversing your sets and reps allows you to do the same number of total repetitions, but increases the average amount of force your muscles apply during the exercise.

Shocking Your Muscles

Cutting your workout in half (below), taking a week off, tri-sets, supersets, and negatives are all different ways to "shock" your muscles so they don't adapt to what you've been doing. As Zig Ziglar says, "If you continue doing what you're doing, you'll continue getting what you've been getting."

Cut your ab workout in half. You may be overtraining your abs. By reducing the demand on them, you'll allow them to recover.

Another option is to take a week off. When you come back stronger after this ab break, you know you were overtrainng.

Tri-sets consist of performing three different exercises for your abs consecutively. Set one is performed, followed immediately by a set of the second and third exercise with no rest in between sets. For example, do a set of crunches followed by side planks on both sides. After completing this tri-set, take a minute break and do the cycle again.

A *superset* is performing two different exercises for your abs and lower back consecutively. Do a set for your back right after a set for your abs. Take no rest between exercises. For example, do a set of reverse crunches followed immediately by bridging. After completing this superset, take a minute break and do the cycle again.

Negatives flex your ab muscles as they lengthen. These are performed by completing a set of an exercise and then having a training partner help you with the up phase of your exercise. If you don't have a partner, use your arms to pull you through the up phase. For example if you were doing crunches, you would grab your legs and pull yourself to the up position. Then perform the down phase unassisted, slowly and with total control.

Reps

Toning your abs is not only achieved by increasing the amount of resistance you are using. Increasing the number of repetitions you perform will make your abs toned and sleek. If you increase the number of repetitions you can do, and maintain perfect form, you have increased your strength and most likely the muscle tone in your abs as well.

But doing hundreds of crunches in a single workout doesn't adequately challenge your muscles. First of all, you are probably not performing perfect crunches, and secondly, if you can do hundreds of crunches with perfect form, you need to add resistance. Doing hundreds of repetitions is similar to chewing gum. You don't get a trimmed, toned jaw if you chew gum.

Adding Resistance

When you train your abs, you damage your muscle fibers. After your workout, your muscle fibers repair—a process that requires calories.

Added resistance to your ab training requires you to use more muscle fibers. You'll increase the number of fibers that are damaged and burn more calories after you've finished your workout.

Increase the weight and do fewer reps (six to eight) if your goal is to gain strength in your abs. Add enough weight to challenge your abs, but not enough to compromise your form.

Do more reps for endurance.

Complete 10 to 12 repetitions with enough resistance to fatigue your muscles if your goal is muscular endurance. Ten reps is a good compromise between absolute strength and muscular endurance.

Rest

Training your abs three days a week is plenty. Figure out which days will work best in your busy schedule. Spread your days out to get enough rest in between your workouts. Tuesday, Thursday, and Saturday works great.

Your Personal Trainer

Don't interlock your fingers behind your head for ab training. You unconsciously pull on your head which decreases your ab work, but increases your chance of neck strain. Instead, place your fingertips lightly behind your ears or cross your arms across your chest.

Rest no longer than a minute between sets.

Short, frequent rest periods during a workout are important so that your abs don't burn out too early in your program. During your rest period, blood delivers oxygen and energy to your abs and carries away waste products.

Rest no longer than a minute between sets of any exercise, though. If you rest too long you may lose "the pump," and decide to call it a day.

In Other Words

Bend your elbow in a "show me your muscle" pose. Blood is forced out of your biceps while your muscle is flexed. After you relax, you feel blood rushing back into your muscle—that is "the pump."

Rest longer on heavy sets and shorter on light sets.

As your conditioning improves, perform the same total number of sets and reps, but lessen your rest periods to a maximum of ten seconds. This requires your muscles to recover faster between sets and increases your results.

The harder the set, the more rest you need. One way to maximize your time is to superset abs and back exercises. For example, do a set of scissors followed immediately by a bridge, and then rest a little longer after the entire superset instead of between each exercise.

Take at least one day of rest between workouts.

Your abdominal muscles should be given 24 to 48 hours of rest before attacking them again. Your muscles firm up between training days. However, too much rest between workouts can hurt your progress. In as little as 72 hours, the benefits of your hard ab-work can begin to disappear.

Chapter **4**

Tone at Home

In This Chapter

- Tone your abs at home
- No equipment necessary
- Engage your abs
- Eliminate love handles

When we're talking about your mid-section, you want less flab and more muscle. Men want their abs rock-hard, ripped, and defined, while women prefer them to be sleek, tight, and flat. Men want to lose their love-handles and women will gladly give away their pooch. Unfortunately, men generally carry extra fat around the waist and women have to deal with the pooch.

This section takes you through your home ab-isolation program. Do these exercises in street clothes. Each exercise only takes 30 seconds. Do 10 repetitions of each exercise. Maintain perfect posture and exhale on the exertion portion of each exercise. Move slowly through each repetition—three seconds up, three seconds down. Never sacrifice your form by trying to get in a few extra reps. Add two repetitions per week until you can perform 20 consecutive repetitions. Below is a quick tour of how to tone at home.

Posture Perfect

Maintain perfect posture and you demonstrate confidence and a balance between your abs and back. Contract your stomach muscles by bringing your navel toward your spine. Imagine a piece of string tied around your waist. If you allow your belly to bulge, the string will break. This is one of the best exercises for making that lower pooch disappear.

Your Personal Trainer

Whether exercising, standing in line, or sitting at your computer, maintaining perfect posture is a great ab exercise.

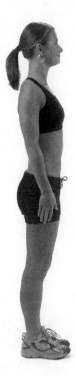

1. Keep your head up, shoulders back, and stomach in.

2. Don't hide your abs, keep your back straight.

Perfect Crunch

Perform the Perfect Crunch and you firm and tone those eye-catching muscles in the front of your stomach. The crunch is the best exercise for targeting all of your abdominal muscles at the same time. Just before you start your crunch, pretend someone is about to hit you in the stomach. Feel your stomach muscles contract and keep using them throughout the duration of your reps. Bring your ribs toward your hips on each rep. Exhale on each rep and draw your navel in toward your spine. Keep your neck in the same position throughout each repetition. Imagine an apple between your chin and your chest. Do not put your hands behind your neck. You will be tempted to start pulling at your neck to get the last few reps, which places unnecessary strain on this fragile part of the spine.

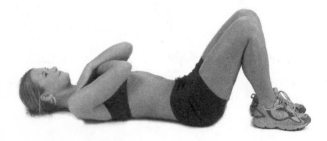

1. Flatten your lower back to the floor and bend your knees to 90 degrees with your feet flat on the floor.

2. Fold your arms across your chest.

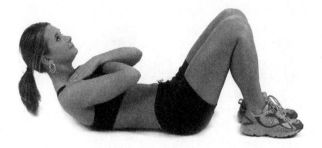

3. As you exhale your breath, curl your chest a couple of inches off of the floor.

4. Hold, then slowly lower your back to the floor and continue your reps.

Get It Right

When you train beyond "the burn" you set yourself up for injury.

Pulsing

Pulsing is a continuous exercise that trains your front ab muscles without resting between reps. Keep your abs flexed for the entire set. Your fingers rest behind your head. They stay open but they do not touch each other. When you interlock your fingers you inadvertently pull on your head. If this exercise is too difficult, cross your arms in front of your chest. If crossing your arms over your chest is too challenging, bring your arms to your side. Exhale through pursed lips during each abbreviated rep.

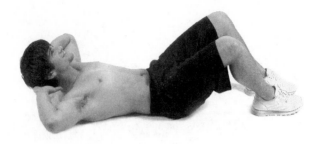

1. Lie on your back with your knees bent and your fingers resting behind your head.

2. Bring your chest toward your knees so that your shoulder blades are just a few inches from the floor.

3. Move about an inch in either direction, pulsing up and down.

Fingers to Toes

Fingers to Toes tones the front of your abs with particular concentration on your upper-ab muscles. It also targets those fingerlike muscles around your ribs. Keep your neck relaxed and don't try to reach too far. If you can keep your hips off of the floor, you'll increase the intensity of the exercise. Exhale during the up phase of each rep as you pull your navel toward your spine. Begin the movement from your abs and not your arms.

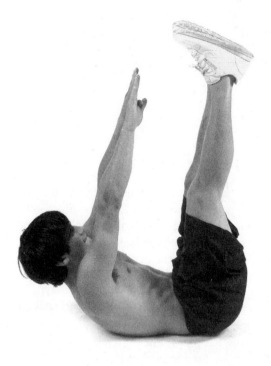

1. Lie on your back with your feet pointed toward the ceiling and your knees straight.

2. Hinge from your waist and extend your fingers toward your toes and raise your hips off of the floor. Keep your back flat to the floor.

3. Lower your hips and shoulders back to the floor.

> **Get It Right**
>
> Your rectus abdominis (six-pack) on the front of your stomach is a single muscle. If you train your lower abs, your upper abs are working, too.

Reverse Crunch

The Reverse Crunch trains the muscles below your naval. Women call this area the pooch—the baby pooch. Firming the muscles in this area helps you to stand taller. Be sure your hips come off of the floor during each repetition. Keep your head and neck resting comfortably on the floor for the entire exercise. Exhale during the up phase of each rep and pull your navel in toward your spine. Maintain a smooth rolling motion for both the up and the down phase. Keep your knees together for the entire exercise. Stop immediately if you have a break in your form.

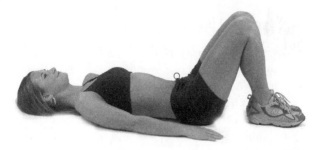

1. Lie on your back with your knees bent and your feet flat on the floor.

2. Keep your arms by your sides.

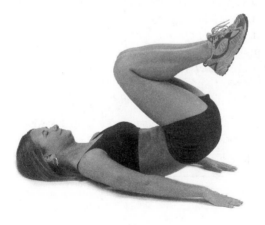

3. Slowly bring your knees toward your chest until your hips come off the floor.

4. Move your knees back until your feet are about an inch from the floor.

Scissors

Scissors is an exercise for the lower abs and side abs. If you had to choose one exercise besides crunches to target your entire abdominal area, this is the one. Your lower back remains on the floor. Exhale through pursed lips on each rep. Draw your navel in toward your spine. Your elbow moves toward your opposite knee and your knee moves toward your opposite elbow in a smooth, reciprocal motion. Maintain flexed abs through the duration of the movement. Keep your hands relaxed (do not pull with your hands) so that your neck doesn't bend forward. When fatigue sets in, be careful not to twist your neck back and forth. If you have a break in your form, stop immediately.

Bet You Didn't Know

The reason we suggest you keep your back flat to the floor and do not recommend maintaining your natural lower back curve is that you might arch your back too much and strain yourself.

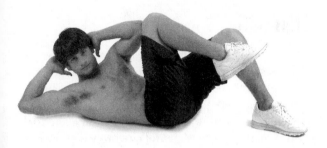

1. Lie on your back with your fingers resting behind your head.

2. Raise your right knee and touch it to your left elbow.

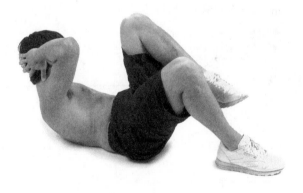

3. Raise your left knee and touch it to your right elbow.

Knee-Ups

Knee-ups are an advanced exercise for your lower abs, almost like a reverse crunch from a vertical position. Since your lower body is working against gravity, this is considered a very advanced exercise. Keep your shoulders down, neck relaxed, head and chest up. Round your back and follow through with your hips so your abs are doing the work. Exhale on each rep and draw your navel in toward your spine. Resist the temptation to swing back and forth. Move very slowly, minimizing momentum. If this exercise is too difficult, try raising one knee at a time.

Get It Right

Train your abs like any other muscle group. Give them at least a day's rest before training them again.

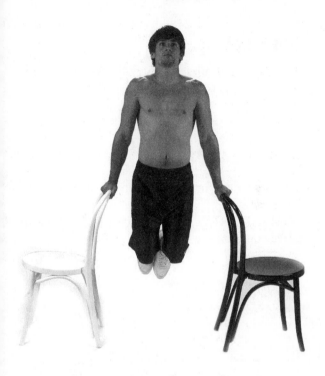

1. Brace yourself between two chairs, elbows slightly bent.

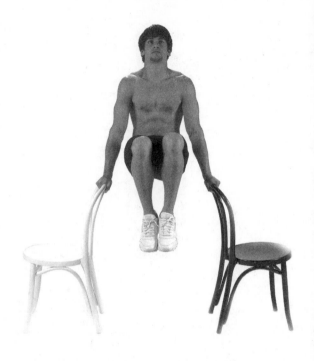

2. Raise your knees toward your chest.

Leg Swings

Leg Swings train the side of your stomach. This is an advanced exercise. The straighter you keep your knees, the harder the exercise. Bend your knees as much as you need to when you first begin doing leg swings. Exhale on each rep and draw your navel in toward your spine. Keep your head and neck relaxed. All movement should begin from your abs.

To increase the intensity, pause for a second at the bottom of each rep. If you feel any lower-back pain, substitute another side-ab exercise for this one.

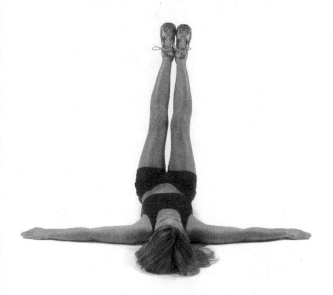

1. Lie on your back with your arms out to your sides.

2. Raise your feet toward the ceiling.

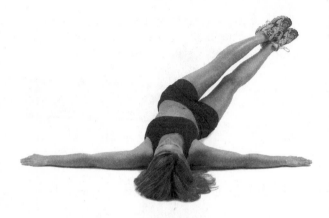

3. Lower your legs to the right until they are five inches from the floor.

4. Repeat on your left side.

Side Abs

Side Abs target the muscles on the sides of your stomach. You may either alternate sides on each repetition or do all of your reps on one side and then all of your reps on the other side. Begin each repetition by flexing your abs. Rest between repetitions if necessary. Keep your neck relaxed. Exhale on each rep and draw your navel in toward your spine. To increase the intensity, bring your fingertips behind your head while your elbows remain out to the side. If this exercise is too difficult, reach your hand toward your opposite knee.

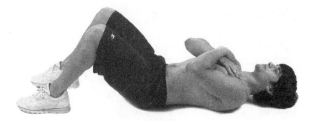

1. Lie on your back with your knees bent.

2. Cross your arms across your chest.

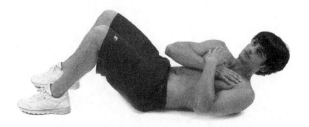

3. Lift your right shoulder toward your left knee.

4. Lift your left shoulder toward your right knee.

Your Personal Trainer

Since you probably do not want the six-pack, rectus abdominis muscles underneath your waistline to grow larger, there is no need to over-train your abs.

The Inside Side Abs

The Inside Side Abs trains muscles on the sides of your stomach and the muscles underneath them. Exhale on each rep and draw your navel in toward your spine. Your head and neck should remain aligned. Although you can't see some of the muscles that are working underneath, they keep your stomach in when you maintain your posture. Don't try to bend too far in either direction when you do this exercise.

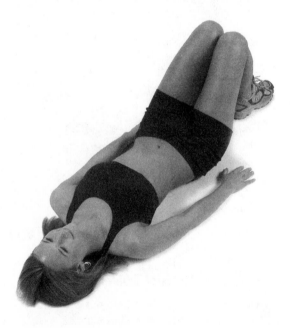

1. Lie on your back with your arms to your sides.

2. Slide your right hand toward your right foot.

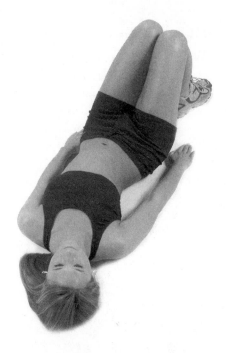

3. Switch sides and repeat.

Chapter 5

Office Abs

In This Chapter

- Tone your abs on the phone
- Exercises without motion
- Target-toning chair workouts
- A stomach to be proud of
- Customized desk workouts

You will be amazed by the results you can achieve by performing simple ab exercises at the privacy of your desk. It's not about sets and reps. You don't need barbells and dumbbells to train your abs. Between phone calls, try the Office Abs routine. Flex your abs while typing on your computer or retrieving your messages.

Hold each movement for three seconds. Begin each exercise by drawing your navel into your spine. Be sure to breathe through each exercise instead of holding your breath. Maintain perfect posture keeping your neck relaxed, chest out, and stomach in. Don't push too hard.

Chair Exercise—Upper Abs

The Chair Exercise—Upper Abs trains your upper stomach muscles. You may do this exercise while talking on the phone or contemplating a decision. Since your abdominal muscles are endurance muscles, do this exercise several times a day; whenever the mood strikes. While you are leaning back, keep your neck in line with your back. Keep your chin up and don't look down towards your chest. Imagine an apple tucked between your chin and your chest.

If this exercise is too difficult, don't lean back all the way to the chair. Instead, lean back until you feel your abs flex. To further tone your abs cross your arms over your chest. And to make this exercise more challenging, place your fingers behind your head in the "TV position." Never interlock your fingers or pull on your head with your hands. Keep your back straight and your head centered directly over your shoulders.

 In Other Words

A **static contraction** is when you squeeze your stomach muscles by holding them flexed without moving.

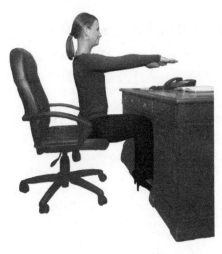

1. Sit on the edge of your chair with your arms extended to the front.

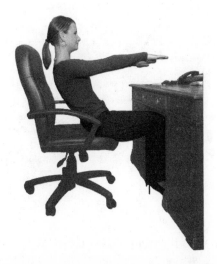

2. Contract your abs and lean back slowly until your upper back touches the back of your chair.

Using Your Desk—Front Abs

Using Your Desk—Front Abs trains the front of your stomach. This exercise strengthens the front abs as well as the top of your leg muscles. Stand up and stretch your legs between sets. Be careful not to press longer than three seconds and don't press too hard. Keep your shoulders back and head up. You may have a tendency to hold your breath during this exercise, so remember to breathe normally. You may also exhale during the exertion phase of each repetition if you prefer. Gradually increase the intensity of each static contraction as you get stronger.

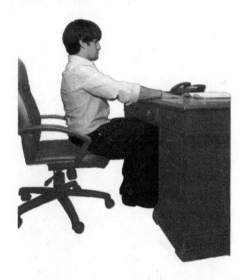

1. Sit in the front of your chair and lift your knees so that they are pressing against the underside of your desk.

2. Place your hands on top of the desk for balance and contract your abs for three seconds, then relax.

Chair Exercise—Front Abs

The Chair Exercise—Front Abs trains the front of your stomach. If you enjoy this exercise, consider trying out for the gymanastics team. Gymnasts have awesome abs and this exercise is one of the reasons why. At first, press your forearms into the chair and unweight your hips from the chair. Keep your knees bent when performing this exercise. No one should detect you are exercising. As your abs get stronger, you may actually be able to lift your hips off of the chair. To challenge yourself further, extend your knees into an "L-Seat." When you can perform an L-Seat, show your colleagues and they will be impressed. Keep your back straight and exhale on each repetition.

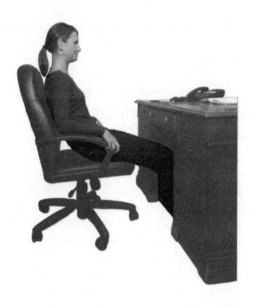

1. Sit in your chair with your back straight and your forearms placed securely on your armrests.

2. Press your forearms into the chair; contract your stomach muscles as if you are lightening the pressure on your seat.

Your Personal Trainer _____

Train your stomach muscles at different angles if you want to see great results.

Chair Exercise–Curls with Resistance

The Chair Exercise—Curls With Resistance trains the front of your stomach and your back. Keep your neck relaxed and your eyes forward. Your arms should remain bent and act as hooks so that they do not fatigue. Flex your abs on the way down and squeeze your abs and back muscles on the way up. Be sure to breathe normally and pay particular attention to your posture. You may exhale on the down phase if you prefer. To make this exercise challenging, add more resistance from your arms.

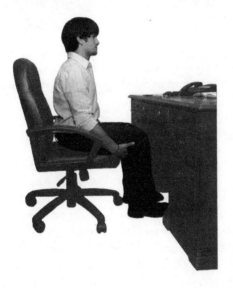

1. Grab underneath your thighs with both hands and curl your chest toward your legs.

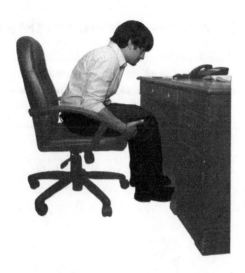

2. Use your arms as resistance as you bring your chest back into your original position.

Chair Exercise—Lower Abs

The Chair Exercise—Lower Abs trains the lower part of your stomach. Be sure to brace your upper body by grabbing the armrests for balance. Raise your feet an inch off of the floor for one second. To add intensity, raise your feet a couple of inches and hold for two seconds. Three inches and three seconds is a very challenging goal to shoot for. If this exercise is too difficult, raise one leg at a time. At first, alternate legs. Then perform all of your reps with one leg, and then all of your reps with the other. This is a very difficult exercise, so start slowly and progress gradually.

The difference between this exercise and Using Your Desk—Front Abs is that on that one you press against the desk as resistance. In Chair Exercise—Lower Abs, the resistance is the weight of your legs, but rather than pressing against the desk you attempt to lift your knees higher than you do on Using Your Desk—Front Abs. This extra range of motion increases the intensity of the exercise.

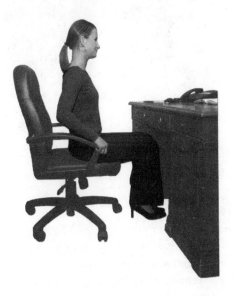

1. Sit perfect posture on the front edge of your chair with your back straight and your neck relaxed.

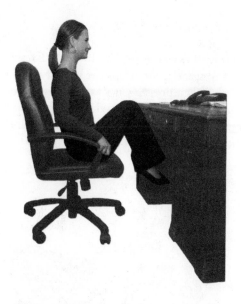

2. Raise your knees toward your chest and then slowly lower them back to the floor.

Bet You Didn't Know

On most stomach exercises, it is very difficult to isolate a certain muscle. All of them work together to get the job done.

Chair Exercise–Side Abs

The Chair Exercise—Side Abs trains the sides of
your stomach. Keep your shoulders down and your
chest out. The first movement you make is to flex
the right side of your stomach closest to your right
arm rest. Do not lean more than a couple of inches,
and think of it as tilting your body sideways from
your waist instead of bending forward. If you perform
it correctly, your office mates shouldn't notice you're
doing this exercise.

Keep your neck relaxed and breathe normally or
exhale on each rep if you prefer. At first, alternate
sides with each rep. To make the exercise more
challenging, perform all of your reps on one side
and then do all of your reps on the other side.

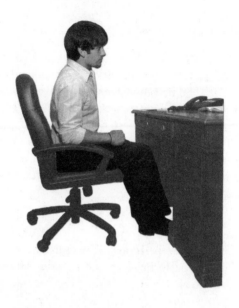

1. Place your right forearm on the armrest and flex the right side of your stomach. Hold for three seconds.

2. Switch sides and repeat.

Chair Exercise—Advanced Side Abs

The Chair Exercise—Advanced Side Abs exercise trains the muscles on the sides of your stomach. Be sure to twist your upper body in the direction of the knee you are lifting. Your knee doesn't have to contact your elbow, so don't bend over more than a couple of inches from your waist. If this exercise is too difficult, bring your hand toward the opposite knee instead of the elbow.

To challenge yourself further on this exercise, place your fingers behind your head and bring your knee toward your opposite elbow. Be sure not to bend your neck and head forward. Raise your knee only slightly at first. As you get stronger, you can raise your knee a few inches on each rep. Breathe normally or exhale on each repetition. This exercise is advanced, so don't try to lift your knee too high too soon.

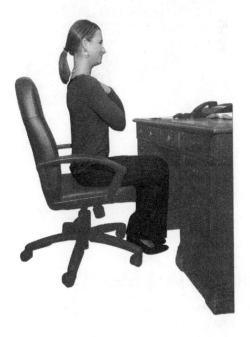

1. Fold your arms across your chest and sit up straight with your feet flat on the floor.

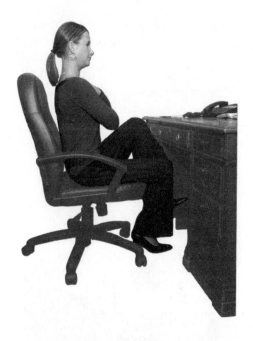

2. Raise your left knee toward your right elbow. Be sure to keep your back straight. Switch sides and repeat.

Using Your Desk–Side Abs

Using Your Desk—Side Abs trains the side of your stomach. This exercise is very simple but it's not easy. Nobody should notice you doing this exercise if you are doing it correctly. Hold each repetition no longer than three seconds. Breathe normally or exhale on each repetition if you prefer. Keep your back straight and alternate sides so you do not

strain the muscles in the tops of your thighs. Use
your armrests for balance.

Although this exercise seems similar to Using
Your Desk—Front Abs, it targets different muscle
groups. When you raise both knees and press them
against the desk you are targeting your lower six-
pack, rectus abdominis. When you raise one knee to
contact your desk, your side abdominal oblique
muscles are the prime movers.

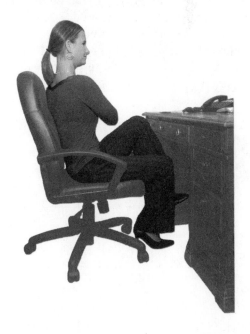

1. Sit on the front edge of your chair and lift
   your right knee so the upper right thigh
   contacts your desk.

2. Switch legs and repeat.

Chair Exercise—Another Side Abs

The Chair Exercise—Another Side Abs exercise tones the sides of your waist from a different angle. Keep your back straight and your neck relaxed. Your head should be aligned with your shoulders. Don't twist too far. Although you may use this move as a stretching exercise, flex your abs to make it a toning workout. At first, alternate sides rather than performing multiple repetitions on the same side. To increase the intensity of this exercise, perform multiple repetitions consecutively on the same side. Be sure to exhale on each repetition. To add a further challenge, let go of the armrest when you feel a maximal contraction of your abs and pause for one second.

Get It Right

Whiplash-type injuries may occur from doing stomach exercises too fast.

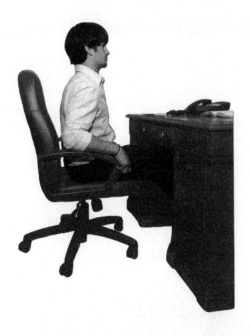

1. Grab the left armrest with your right hand. Twist to your left and flex the left side of your stomach for three seconds.

2. Grab the right armrest with your left hand. Twist to your right and flex the side of your stomach for three seconds.

Chair Exercise—Advanced Side Abs

Chair Exercise—Advanced Side Abs trains the muscles on the sides of your stomach. Be careful not to lean your body too far to the side. Keep your back straight between reps. To increase the intensity of this exercise, place your fingers behind your head. Do not pull on your head with your hands. Exhale through each repetition. It is extremely important not to bend your neck, instead tilt from your waist.

To add a further challenge, when you feel a maximal contraction of your abs pause for a one-second count.

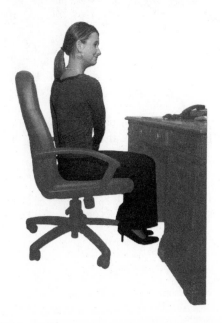

1. Cross your arms over your chest and keep your back straight, stomach in, and chest out.

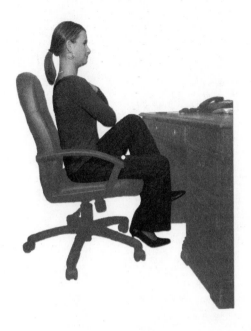

2. Tilt your upper body to the right while lifting your right knee toward that elbow.

3. Tilt your upper body to the left while lifting your left knee toward that elbow. Don't try to bend too far.

Chapter 6

Tone and Tighten

In This Chapter

- Incredible, gym-toned abs
- Form first, no midsection bulge
- Tighten your waistline
- Weights work, your program grows with you

Home and office training is fine, but training your abs in the gym will get you to the next level. It's nice to be in the company of like-minded people. Some people go to the gym simply to be inspired by hard bodies they admire. Be careful, however, of the well-meaning wannabe bodybuilder attempting to share his latest ab-blasting workout. Take your Pocket Idiot's Guides to the gym and compare his suggestions to our tried-and-true methods.

There is nothing like "feeling the burn" on that tenth rep. Maintain perfect form on every exercise. Move through a full range of motion, paying particular attention to keeping your neck relaxed. Depending on the exercise, your lower back should either be pressed to the floor or in its natural curve. Begin each exercise by using your lower abdominal muscles to draw your navel toward your spine. Continue to flex these muscles through the duration of each repetition. If you cannot perform 10 repetitions with perfect form, decrease the amount of weight you are using. Breathe normally at first, but when the going gets tough, exhale on the exertion part of each repetition. When you can perform 10 repetitions with perfect form, it's time to add a couple pounds of resistance.

Seated Crunches with Resistance Bands

Seated Crunches with Resistance Bands trains the front of your stomach. The added resistance from the bands firm and tone your muscles. Anchor the exercise band securely. Concentrate on flexing your abs at the beginning of your rep. Keep tension on your abs throughout the duration of your set without resting in the up or down position. Move very slowly through each rep: three seconds down, three seconds up. Keep your elbows tucked into your body. Be careful not to pull with your arms. Sit with perfect posture between each rep. Round your back on each repetition. Curl your chest toward your legs. As your stomach muscles get stronger, add more resistance.

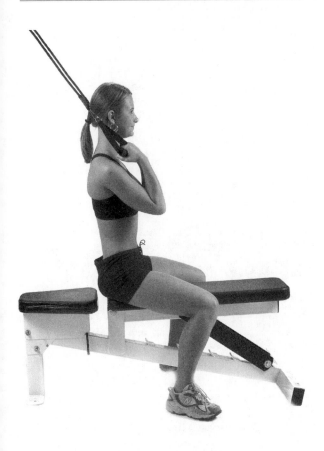

1. Begin in a seated position holding the handles of your resistance bands at neck level. The bands attach to the wall above head level.

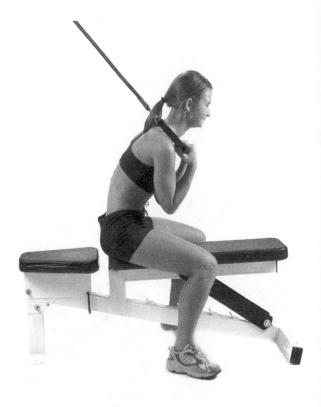

2. Lean forward from your waist until you reach a 45 degree angle. As you exhale, keep your back straight and your chin off of your chest.

3. Return to your starting position and complete your repetitions.

In Other Words

Besides your six-pack, the muscles on the sides of your stomach (external and internal obliques) and your coughing muscle (transverse abdominis) are important for every move you make.

Front Plank

Front Plank trains all of your stomach muscles and your back as well. Be sure to keep your back straight and neck relaxed. Your back and neck will have a tendency to sag. Hold for three seconds. If you have a break in your form, stop the exercise immediately. Add two sets per week until you can perform ten sets of three-second reps consecutively. At first, rest as long as you need to between sets. As you get stronger and develop more endurance, decrease the rest time between sets. Be sure to breathe normally during each repetition. If this exercise is too difficult, do it from your knees instead of your feet.

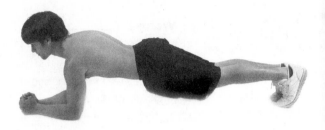

1. Start from your hands and knees and then slowly drop to your forearms and the balls of your feet. Keep your elbows in line with your shoulders. And some people like to clasp their hands together making a triangle, rather than fingertips facing forward.

2. Contract your stomach and back muscles, but keep the rest of your body relaxed.

Shoulder Bridge

Shoulder Bridge trains your stomach and back muscles. This is a great exercise to do on the floor while watching TV. Keep your feet hip-width apart. Your heels should be directly under your knees, your arms to your side. Pull your navel toward your spine and, without arching your back, lift your hips toward the ceiling. Your body should form a straight, slanted line from your knees to your chest. Hold the bridge position for three seconds. Add two sets per week until you can perform ten sets of three-second reps consecutively. Your neck and shoulders should be straight. Imagine you have an apple between your chin and your chest. At first, rest as long as you need to between sets. As you get stronger and develop more endurance, decrease the rest time between sets. Be sure to breathe normally during each repetition. If you prefer, you may exhale during the rep. Keep your hips elevated and level throughout the duration of the exercise.

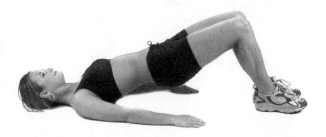

1. Lie down on your back with your knees bent and your arms to the side. Press with your heels to lift yourself into the bridge or ramp position.

2. Keep your neck relaxed and your back straight.

Your Personal Trainer

For every exercise you do for your stomach, do two for your back. Fortunately, most of the exercises in this chapter train your back as well as your stomach so that you will maintain perfect balance and symmetry.

Roll Up

The Roll Up trains the muscles in the front of your stomach. This is a fun exercise you can do with your kids. It is relatively easy to do, so you may perform more than ten reps if you wish. It's a great warm-up or cool-down exercise for your abs. Roll as slowly as you can, three seconds in both directions minimizes momentum. Be sure you are rolling on a mat or thick carpet. Keep your chin tucked to your chest and be careful not to roll too far in either direction.

Have fun with this one.

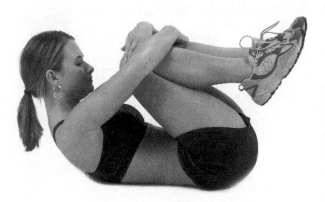

1. Lie on your back with your knees tucked into your chest.

2. Wrap your arms around your legs and begin rolling back and forth.

Butterfly Crunch

The Butterfly Crunch trains the muscles in the front of your stomach. Although this exercise looks kind of funny, it's awesome for your abs. You place the soles of your feet together to keep your upper-leg muscles from helping your abs out. Since your legs can't help, your abs are doing all of the work. Keep your back flat on the floor and begin each rep by contracting your stomach muscles. Curl your chest a couple of inches toward your legs on each repetition.

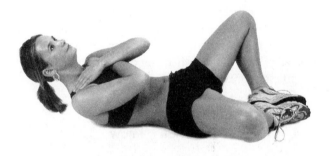

1. Lie on your back with your arms crossed over your chest.

2. Place the soles of your feet together as close to your body as possible with your knees bent.

3. Imagine you have an apple tucked between your chin and your chest and raise your shoulder blades a few inches off the floor.

4. Hold, then lower your back slowly to the floor.

Twists with Resistance Bands

Twists with resistance bands train the sides of your stomach. This is a great exercise to firm and tone your entire waistline. These muscles are necessary for your daily activities, so the stronger the better. As your flexibility improves, you may twist a little further. Anchor the exercise band securely. Be sure to maintain perfect posture throughout the duration of each rep. Do not bend over from the waist. Move slowly and purposefully. Three seconds in both directions works great. Don't attempt to twist too far.

Perform ten repetitions with perfect form. For a further challenge, as you get stronger, you may double the exercise band to add more resistance. Only add resistance when you can perform ten reps without a break in your form.

Bet You Didn't Know

If you miss a workout, no sweat. It is not one workout that matters, it is the weeks and months of training that make a difference.

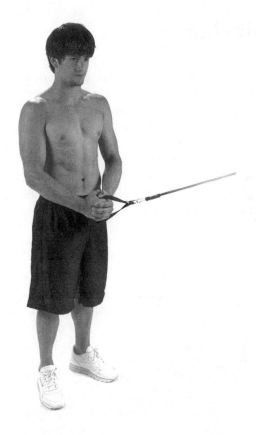

1. Stand with your feet shoulder-width apart and your knees slightly bent. Hold the resistance band beside your waist.

2. Contract the sides of your stomach as you gently turn to the right. When you feel the contraction, stop and return to your original position.

3. Switch sides and repeat.

Side Planks

Side Planks train the sides of your stomach and lower-back muscles at the same time. Be sure to keep your body straight (don't sag) and hold for three seconds. If this exercise is too challenging from your feet, try it from the outside of your calf. If that is still too hard, do it from the side of your hip. Add two sets per week until you can perform ten sets of three-second reps consecutively. At first, rest as long as you need to between sets. As you get stronger and develop more endurance, decrease the rest time between sets. Be sure to breathe normally during each repetition, or, if you prefer, you may exhale throughout the rep. You may decide to alternate right and left side planks to save time. As you get stronger, decrease the time between sets, and perform all of your planks on one side and then all of your planks on the other side.

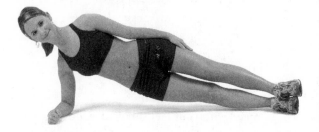

1. Lie on your side bracing your body with your forearm and the outside edge of your shoe.

2. Lift your hip off of the floor and hold your body straight.

3. Switch sides and repeat.

Reverse Crunches with Resistance Bands

Reverse Crunches with Resistance Bands train the lower part of your stomach underneath your navel (the pooch). Anchor the exercise band securely. Perform ten repetitions with perfect form. Move three seconds in both directions. As your abs get stronger, add more resistance by doubling up on the band. As you add more resistance, work your way back up to ten reps. Be sure to lift your hips off the floor at the end of each rep so that your legs are not doing the work that your abs are supposed to do.

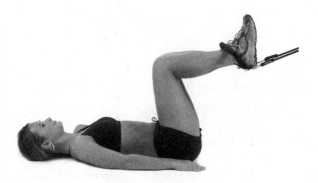

1. Lie on your back with your knees bent and the resistance bands anchored to your ankles. Keep your arms to your side.

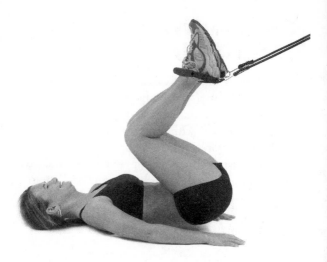

2. Raise your knees toward your chest until
   your hips leave the floor.

Reverse Crunches with Weights on Your Legs

Reverse Crunches with Weights on Your Legs tones
the muscles of the lower pooch. Since gravity and
stability are involved, you will be training other
balancing muscles in your abs as well. Be sure the
weights are secured to your legs. Don't try to lift
too much too soon or you'll strain your upper-leg
muscles. Since you are using weights instead of
resistance bands, there will be a tendency for you to
use momentum. Three seconds in both directions
minimizes inertia.

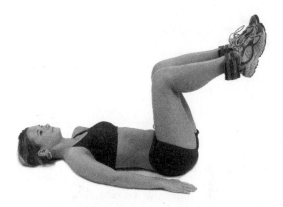

1. Lie on your back with your knees bent and ankle weights resting on the top of your ankles. Place your arms to your sides.

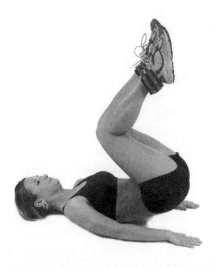

2. Lift your knees toward your chest, using your arms to balance until your hips leave the floor.

Get It Right

Momentum is your worst enemy in the weight room. Move slowly to prevent injury and to be sure the correct muscles are working.

Leg Raise

The Leg Raise tones the lower part of your stomach. Begin with your legs pointing straight up in the air with your knees slightly bent. Slowly lower your legs toward the floor. To prevent lower-back pain, be sure your lower back is flat to the floor. If you have never done this exercise before, bend your knees at 90 degrees. Find a range of movement that is comfortable, and be sure that your lower back does not come off of the floor. If your lower back begins to arch, do not let your legs drop any further. To prevent arching your back, you can tuck your hands underneath your rear end, and this will help keep your back flat.

Continue doing reps, beginning with your feet pointing toward the ceiling and then slowly lowering them. Three seconds up, three seconds down. Always stay in a range of motion where your back does not arch. Do these for ten reps. Keep your neck relaxed through each rep. Breathe normally on this exercise. As you get stronger, you may extend your knees a little. Never fully extend your knees.

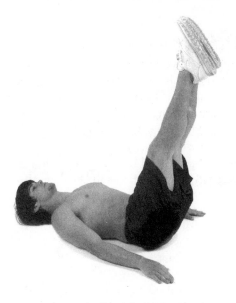

1. Lie on your back with your arms to your side and your knees slightly bent.

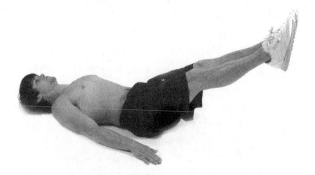

2. Lift your legs toward the ceiling and lower them very slowly a few inches.

3. Return them to the starting position.

Leg Push

The Leg Push works the lower part of your stomach. Although it is a very small movement, be sure to maintain perfect form so that your lower-stomach muscles are working. If you cannot complete the three-second rep, begin with one-second reps. Add a second to each rep each week until you can perform ten three-second reps. Be sure to breathe throughout each repetition and keep your back straight and neck relaxed.

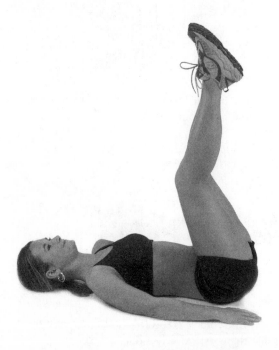

1. Lie on your back with your arms to your sides and your feet pointed toward the ceiling.

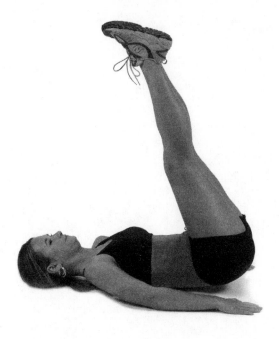

2. Flex your lower abdominal muscles so that your hips lift off of the floor for three seconds.

Chapter 7

Incinerate Fat

In This Chapter

- Accelerate fat loss
- Multi-task ab exercises
- Stretching your abs and back
- One-minute-a-day workouts
- All you need in one package

Losing fat around your waist is easier than liposuction. You don't have to train until you're breathless or stay at a certain pace on the treadmill. You burn fat all day long. Little movements use energy and burn fat. Standing up and stretching, walking your dog, walking to the refrigerator—all incinerate fat. Figure out ways to add more movement into your day. The more you move, the better.

This chapter teaches you to lose fat the easy way. Choose your favorite fat-burning moves. One way to shed fat all day long is to flex your muscles. That's right, flex your abs whenever you think of it. Toned abs are rock-hard instead of flabby. Your abs will get firmer through conscious effort. If you keep your abs flexed they'll tend to stay firmer longer. Flexed abs use up more energy than relaxed abs. When your abs are flexed, there is more cross-bridging between your actin and myosin filaments. The small strands (actin) and large strands (myosin) in your muscle fibers are pulled together by cross-bridges. The more cross-bridging that's happening, the more chiseled and toned your abs are.

Your Favorite Sitcom Is Your Workout

Work out while you watch your favorite TV show. In a 30-minute program there are five minutes of commercials for you to move. In a two-hour program there are about 25 minutes of commercials. Simply get off of the couch during each commercial and move.

A safe and effective way to train the front of your stomach while watching TV is the ubiquitous crunch. But to do a perfect crunch you have to maintain perfect form. The first part of the crunch is to flatten your lower back to the floor.

Put your hands on your abs to feel them work during the crunch. The crunch is a very small movement, and to others it might look like you're just goofing off and doing incomplete reps. But when summer comes, you'll be able to show them your sleek and chiseled six-pack.

You can get the most out of your stomach muscle exercises by bending your hips and knees to reduce the action of your hip flexors and to protect your lower back.

Placing your thighs at a right angle to your torso to begin with means that the hip flexors can't pull the torso any further, so more of the work is done by your abs instead of your legs.

With your feet flat on the floor, press down and back with your heels. By pressing your heels into the floor you activate your hamstring muscles in the back of your leg. This keeps your hip flexor muscles from taking over for your abs.

> **Bet You Didn't Know**
>
> It doesn't take 20 minutes of exercise to begin burning fat around your waist. Break your workouts into a few minutes each, scattered throughout your day.

Indoor Training

A quick warm-up helps you burn more fat during your cardio. Do five minutes of ab-isolation exercises as your warm-up.

Choose any type of cardio you wish. You may use all of the different exercise machines or be creative by running around your house. You can jog up the stairs, skip through your hallways, and dance in your living room.

You might try walking in place while you watch your favorite TV show—who needs a treadmill anyway? If that's too easy, step up and down on a low bench. Stepping is harder, but it burns more stomach fat.

Chores are workouts too. Every movement that you do begins from your abs. Find the most vigorous chores you can handle. Your significant other will be very happy with the new you.

Next time you are doing the dishes take notice that your abs are tight. Whether you are cleaning the counter or returning a milk jug to the refrigerator you're training your abs.

 Your Personal Trainer

Your body adapts to training, so change up your workout program occasionally.

Outdoor Training

If you have a yard there is no need to spend hours in the gym training your abs. Next time you rake leaves or sweep your driveway, focus on the toning effect on the sides of your stomach. When you lean to the side and pull, you are getting a great ab-isolation workout.

Stretching Your Abs

General stretching is good for both your body and your brain. Blood flow is stimulated to increase your energy level. Through regular, active stretching, you will feel a greater sense of well-being, far greater vitality, and a calmer, more-relaxed attitude.

Stretching improves the elasticity of your abdominal muscles and ligaments surrounding your joints. It improves flexibility and helps to prevent injury and soreness. Stretching promotes muscular balance and relaxation and also decreases the resistance of your tissues.

For safety, never stretch a cold muscle. On warm days you can touch your toes; on cooler days you barely reach your knees. You can hold your stretch more comfortably in the afternoon than in the morning. Go for comfort. Settle into your pose. Breathe deeply from your diaphragm. Exhale as you move into each position. Hold your stretch at least 10 seconds in order to fully relax the muscle. Breathe normally between each stretch; take deep breaths from your diaphragm and exhale into each stretch to nourish your muscles and aid in relaxation. Add two seconds a week until you work up to 30 seconds. Within months you may stretch to a slight level of tension but never approaching pain.

Get It Right

Bouncing into your stretch may cause micro-tears in your muscles. So instead of bouncing, relax and breathe into your stretch.

C-Stretch

The C-Stretch elongates your stomach muscles. Keep your neck aligned with your head and your shoulders down. Exhale into the deeper part of your stretch, but otherwise breathe normally. Be careful not to stretch too fast or too far. Stretch until you feel tension and then stop. If you are very flexible, you may extend the stretch by moving from your forearms to your hands. Press your hands into the floor and slowly extend your elbows until you feel tension. Always warm up before you stretch.

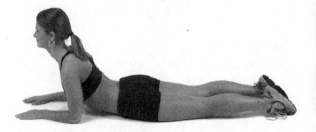

1. Lie on your stomach with your forearms under your shoulders and your palms on the floor.

2. Press your forearms into the floor as you raise your upper body, stretching from your waist. Hold for 30 seconds.

Upper-Thigh Stretch

The Upper-Thigh Stretch lengthens the muscles in the upper-front part of your leg called the hip flexors. Begin in a lunge position with your front leg bent at 90 degrees and your back leg straight. Keep your back straight and neck relaxed. Lean into your front leg. Be careful that your knee does not travel over your toe. Lean your upper body back slightly, tilting your pelvis forward. Breathe normally, but exhale into the deep part of the stretch.

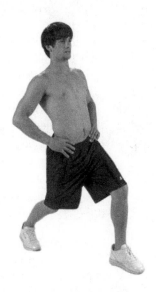

1. Stand with your left knee bent and your right leg straight behind you.

2. Tilt your pelvis forward and hold the stretch for 30 seconds.

Your Personal Trainer

Hold your stretch for 30 seconds to combat the myotatic response or stretch reflex. The stretch reflex is the rubber band–like recoil that you feel when you stretch a muscle too far too fast.

Lower-Back Flex

The Lower-Back Flex stretches out your lower back. If you do not bend down and bring your knees to your chest occasionally, you will lose the flexibility to perform this exercise. Many people from other countries possess outstanding flexibility because they squat in this position several hours a day. If this exercise puts too much pressure on your knees, you may do it from a side-lying position.

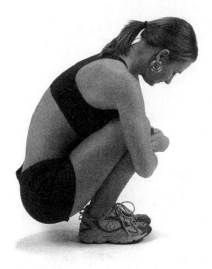

1. Squat on the floor with your knees to your chest.

2. Wrap your arms around your legs and bring your chin to your chest. Hold for 30 seconds.

Lower-Back Arch

The Lower-Back Arch stretches all of the muscles in your back. You probably sit at your desk all day, sit at meals, and then sit for your morning and evening drive. The front of your body tightens up in this flexed position. To combat short, tight muscles, stretch them in the opposite direction. Keep your neck in line with your spine. Maintain a stable base by keeping your knees slightly bent. Perform this exercise several times a day. Do not lean back too far. Be sure to keep your head up to maintain your balance.

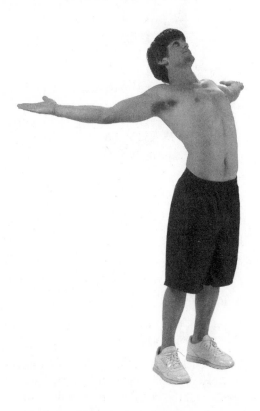

1. Stand with your feet shoulder-width apart and your arms out to the side.

2. Lean back with your chest high and hold for 30 seconds.

Back-of-Leg Stretch

The Back-of-Leg Stretch loosens up the muscles in the back of your upper leg. This exercise may be done while you are at work or if you are waiting in line. Perform this exercise several times a day to help keep your posture perfect. Stretching the backs of your legs also helps to prevent lower-back pain. Keep your back straight and your head up. Maintain a slight arch in your lower back with your hips back. Place both hands on the middle thigh of your supporting right leg.

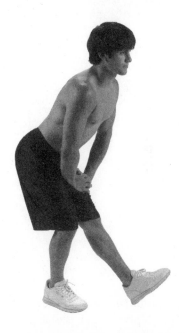

1. Stand with your feet shoulder-width apart and your weight on your right leg. Keep your right knee bent.

2. Extend your left knee, hinge at the hip, and feel a stretch in the back of your left leg. Hold this stretch for 30 seconds.

3. Switch sides and repeat.

Chapter 8

Flab to Fab

In This Chapter

- ◆ Better body eating system
- ◆ Eat more, weigh less
- ◆ Short-on-time meals
- ◆ Nutritious living

To get rid of stubborn abdominal fat, eating right is essential. You must lose that layer of fat between the skin and the muscle to see those abs. This eating program is designed to do just that.

You may have tried one diet after another with no long-term success. You stopped eating carbohydrates and noticed a rapid weight loss. This looked and felt okay at first, but in a short time, water-weight returned and you still couldn't see your abs.

How Diets Work

After a month or so on a low-carb diet, you were blindsided by a pizza commercial. You decided to eat just one slice and save the leftovers. The last thing you remember was devouring the entire pizza and thinking, "I blew it, so I might as well finish this carton of ice cream, too." You fell off the wagon, gained your stomach back—and a few pounds more.

At first you might lose weight on a low-carb diet, but the loss of muscle and resulting metabolic slow-down causes you to regain your gut. And contrary to what your friends at the gym say, doing sit-ups while starving yourself isn't the answer, either.

Bet You Didn't Know

Low-carb diets restrict fruits, vegetables, and whole grains, and they are tough to stay on.

It's easy to follow a step-by-step plan of cabbage or grapefruit and lose weight. The weight you lose is fat, muscle, and water; probably not in that order.

There are calorically dense carbs and nutrient-dense carbs. Calorically dense carbs are foods such as pasta, bagels, and boxed cereals—a lot of calories in a small serving. Nutrient-dense carbohydrates energize your muscles for the long haul. These include fruits, veggies, and whole grains.

If you're a marathon runner or ultra-distance cyclist, you burn up extra calories. But if you work a desk job and don't have the time to run, bike, or swim several hours a day, eat nutrient-dense carbs.

Nutrient-dense carbs don't add inches to your stomach—eating too many calories does. If you eat more than you burn, regardless of the source of those calories (carbohydrates, proteins, or fats), your love handles grow.

Protein is a necessary nutrient to chisel those abs. Eat a serving of protein about the size of a deck of cards at each meal. Protein is muscle-building fuel as long as you eat enough carbs. If you eat enough nutrient-dense carbs, that allows protein to do its job to tone those abs. If you eat too few carbs, the protein you eat has no choice but to be used for energy.

Whether you get your protein from beef, pork, chicken, or turkey, go for the leaner cuts. If you are a vegetarian, eat low-fat dairy, tofu, and lots of beans and legumes.

Even the leanest animal protein contains fat, and eating too much saturated fat is not heart-healthy. The solution is to eat the right kind of fat. Garnish your meat, fruits, and veggies with healthy omega-three monounsaturated and unsaturated fats. Nuts, seeds, and peanut butter are also tasty, ab-chiseling essential fats. Eat fish several days a week. Fish is rich in omega-three fat and ab-sculpting protein.

Your Personal Trainer

Diet sodas don't satisfy a craving. If you miss the potato chip crunch, choose cauliflower, broccoli, peppers, carrots, or celery.

Eat to Fuel Your Muscles

Your mother taught you to eat fruits and vegetables. Add a portion of lean protein with a tablespoon of your favorite healthy essential fat and you're on the program.

Think of a round plate cut in thirds. One third is a lean protein, one third is a fruit, and one third is a vegetable.

And don't forget water. Drink about 64 ounces of water a day. But if you work out hard, drink more than that. If it's dry and hot, or if you are sweating profusely, drink liberally. Water by itself won't chisel those abs, but it keeps your metabolism revved.

The first and most important change you can make is to limit your soft drink consumption. Drink water instead of soft drinks. The average can of your favorite beverage contains about 10 teaspoons of sugar. Replace sugared drinks immediately and within a couple of weeks you will see changes in your body.

Three things happen to the calories that you eat. Either they are burned up by your metabolism or activity, stored in your muscle, or stored as fat. Try eating small meals throughout the day instead of a couple of large ones. Your fat cells are a lot less likely to fill up if you eat mini-meals because your body has immediate energy to draw from. If you eat large quantities of food in a single sitting, your body stores what it doesn't need at the moment. And yes, your body will store this extra energy as fat. A few hours later, you will be hungry again, even though your fat stores are full.

Spend a few minutes each evening planning the next day's meals and snacks. If you know what you're going to eat, you won't find yourself ravenous at the counter of a fast-food restaurant.

In Other Words

The Thermic Effect of Food (TEF) means that when you eat, your body expends calories digesting and assimilating your food.

Use the eating-frequency plan that works best for you and your particular lifestyle. A mid-morning mini-meal helps stabilize blood sugar so you won't be ravenous at lunch, but if you eat a huge breakfast of eggs, whole-wheat toast, and oatmeal, you may not need a snack between breakfast and lunch.

Eat until you're full or you'll be back for more. If your body hasn't received enough nutrients it'll let you know.

When you eat food your body must work hard to digest it. When your body works hard it uses up calories. Eating breakfast-snack-lunch-snack-dinner keeps your metabolism revved all day long. You are constantly feeding your muscle so you don't have to worry about muscle being used for energy.

Give our eating program a chance. It takes a few weeks to go from fast-food flab to fab abs. Eat tasty foods but prepare them correctly. Unlike bland, tasteless health food, this program is a combination of delicious and ab-friendly foods that you can eat anytime, anywhere. If you crave a burger and fries, brown the hamburger meat and rinse it in hot water before you grill it. Broil your fries in the oven and you have created a better choice. Eating lean is as appetizing as your creativity. It is in the preparation. Make better choices if you are forced to eat fast food. Lean more toward salads and grilled or baked foods that many restaurants offer now.

Choose skim milk instead of regular, mustard on sandwiches instead of mayonnaise, low-calorie frozen desserts instead of ice cream, and use low-calorie salad dressing.

Several factors determine how many calories you burn during your workout. If you are bigger, you incinerate more calories than a smaller person. The harder you work, the more your waistline will shrink. If it is extremely cold or hot, your body burns extra calories to maintain your normal temperature. And if you are fit, you burn more abdominal fat than a sedentary person, even in your sleep.

Your muscles are 70 percent water. Before you begin your training, drink two cups of water. To keep your ab muscles full and tight, begin drinking six ounces of water every 20 minutes throughout your workout.

A variety of sports drinks are available. Sometimes these drinks are too sugary, so you may decide to dilute them with water. If your sports drink is too tasty, it might slosh around too long in your stomach.

Sports drinks that contain more than 7 percent carbohydrate are absorbed slower than those with less sugar.

Include a little protein in your after-workout snack. Working out tears down muscle tissue. Protein rebuilds muscle. Pair a tuna-on-whole-wheat with that glass of juice.

How much you eat before and after your workout depends on your activity level and your metabolism. Try having a snack before your workout and see if that helps you move a little further or get a few extra reps.

The more you work out and the harder each workout is, the more food you need. If you walk a mile, that burns about 100 calories. If you take an indoor cycling class, count on burning at least 450 calories. There are all kinds of formulas to try and determine how many calories you should eat, depending on your metabolism.

If you are moderately active—you walk 30 minutes 4 days a week, and lift weights twice a week—then multiply your body weight by 13. The number you came up with equals the minimum number of calories you should eat each day just to support your metabolism.

Keeping a food journal will help keep track of how many calories you are really getting. Writing everything down will help you keep track of your protein, carb, and fat intake. You may find that you are not getting enough of one thing and too much of another.

Get It Right _____

Have soup as an appetizer. You will eat less during your meal.

Eat to Starve Your Fat Cells

At first, you have to walk a tightrope between not eating too much and not eating enough. If you eat too much, the extra calories will be stored around your midsection. If you don't eat enough, your body will hold on to fat and use your muscles for energy.

Experiment with your eating program until you notice that your waistline is getting smaller and your abs are tighter. If you continue the program and add muscle to your body, the metabolic increase will allow you to eat more food without gaining fat.

Nobody eats right 100 percent of the time. If you deprive yourself of a certain type of food, you will want it more. Rather than eat all of the health food in your house and then succumb to the "forbidden" item, go ahead and satisfy your craving immediately. On the other hand, if you know that a "trigger food" will set off a binge, don't start. The best way to eliminate trigger foods is to not have them in your home.

You will know if the eating program is working. Your energy level will be up and your pants will be looser. There is no need to get your body fat checked or buy an expensive scale.

Eat for the right reasons. Most people eat for reasons other than hunger. For one month, develop the mentality that you're going to eat to fuel your workouts. After a month, do what you like. You'll be amazed at the difference this makes in how you approach eating.

Think of food as a fuel instead of a treat. Sure, you should enjoy all of your meals, but if you can change your mind about food, you will be rewarded with great abs.

Other factors in your life will also contribute to losing fat around those abs. Be sure you are getting enough sleep and handling stress. Too much stress tends to deposit fat just where you don't want it: on those abs.

Success on your eating program might require you to pre-prepare your foods. Choose a day of the week where you can grill your favorite foods and prepare casseroles to store in the fridge or to freeze. If you are really organized, you could plan a monthly menu.

Although professional athletes may weigh their food and actors endorse pre-packaged diets, be careful not to obsess about your eating. Any worthwhile program takes time. You might see results quickly. But if not, be patient and you will have your abs.

Chapter 9

Your Total Program

In This Chapter

- ◆ Small changes get great abs
- ◆ Eat, Exercise, Commit
- ◆ Flatten your stomach the easy way
- ◆ Attack fat
- ◆ Putting your workout program together

You want your stomach to have a firmer, more-compact appearance. Women especially may find that their lower pooch is a storage site for considerable excess fat.

Unfortunately, just exercising your stomach muscles won't accomplish "spot reduction." During any type of exertion, fat is mobilized from all of your storage deposits equally, not just those near the exercising muscles. The best exercise to reduce fat in the lower stomach is general activity.

If a 20-minute boot camp class in the gym is too much to ask, do 5-minute mini-workouts throughout the day. Less is best when seeking better abs. It's better to do some easy activity for 5 minutes every hour than to be sedentary all day and take a 20-minute aerobic class in the evening. Besides, you have to drive to the studio and spend time showering afterwards. If you can't get to the gym, do our office ab-isolation exercises. If your job requires you to travel, do your ab exercises on the plane or in a taxi. Make up your mind to remain consistent and you will see results.

Bet You Didn't Know

You are burning fat all of the time. Using up your fat stores is a cumulative effort. You don't have to be working out for 20 minutes straight to burn fat.

Increase Your Activity

You are burning calories while you sit. If you stand you burn more calories. You burn even more calories if you walk, jog, or run (in that order). The more calories you burn, the more fat you lose, but you don't have to work out hard to minimize your waistline. Puttering works. Treat your yard work or household chores as your workout.

Your new set of activities should leave you energized with a feeling of accomplishment. Your movement should be challenging but not painful. If you feel exhausted, you trained too hard.

Move an Extra 20 Minutes a Day

You may decide to use a pedometer that attaches to your belt like a pager. It keeps track of how many steps you take each day. Aim for about 10,000 steps a day.

Although you have probably heard these suggestions before, they really work. Shedding fat around your waist is a cumulative effort.

Train yourself to move instead of being still. Be creative about adding movement into your day. When your exercise is a pleasure, developing those abs will be easy.

Add Five Minutes a Week to Your Activity

Twenty minutes of extra activity goes a long way toward seeing those abs, but don't stop there. Add 5 minutes each week to see even better results. In just 4 weeks you will be moving 40 minutes a day more than you were before. That extra activity pays dividends toward chiseling those abs.

The more you move, the higher your energy level. With increased energy, you move more. It's a cycle of progress that trims your abs in no time.

In Other Words

Crossing your anaerobic threshold or lactate threshold means that you are no longer training at a steady state. You have crossed over the line and are huffing and puffing and burning.

Move Fast or Move Slow—Just Move

It doesn't matter how fast you step, walk, jog, or pedal. Move at your own pace and breathe effortlessly. Every once in a while, when you're feeling peppy, pick up the pace a little.

Remember, though, the most important aspect of your activity program is that it should be easy. If you try to do too much too soon, it is no longer easy.

By taking baby steps, there should be no discomfort. As your conditioning gradually improves, you will want to challenge yourself by speeding up.

Speed up just enough so that if you go faster you'll be a little breathless. If you lose your breath, slow down. Truly enjoy every second of your activity. It is not about huffing and puffing and burning.

Accessories Make the Workout

Before you progress, be sure you're dressed properly. Comfortable, supportive, breathable clothes are important to continue melting fat. The most important part of your exercise wardrobe is your shoes. If your feet don't feel good, you'll find a reason to stop moving. Check with your nearest athletic footwear store and get your feet sized and fitted for a pair of shoes with the correct support and cushioning. Also wear comfortable, breathable clothing.

Another crucial factor in accelerating your fat loss is motivation. Exercise feels easier when you listen to music. Moving to the beat of your favorite artist is exhilarating. Listening to music while pedaling a stationary bike or walking on a treadmill inspires

you to work out longer and harder. If you train out-
doors, keep your headphones turned down so you
can hear approaching dogs or cars.

Now You're Really Moving

After you can successfully move for 25 consecutive
minutes try this: Following your warm-up, walk,
pedal, or step very slowly for 10 seconds. Then pick
up the pace for the next 10 seconds. Drop back to
your original slow movement for 10 seconds. Repeat
this slow-fast 10-second cycle for 10 minutes. Con-
gratulations! You have just completed your first
interval workout.

Intervals bump up the intensity of your activity, which
burns more total calories. You also continue burning
more calories after your interval workout is over.

The longer and more intense you work out, the
greater the after-burn. That is, while you are showering and sitting on your couch, you continue to
burn extra calories from your workout.

On all of the interval activity programs below, be
sure to warm up and cool down for 5 minutes. Warm-
ing up and cooling down is moving slowly. Begin
with easy movement, and then gradually increase
the pace. Moving fast simply means moving at a
pace that is challenging but doable.

Program 1: After your warm-up, move at about 70
percent of your maximum effort for 15 seconds. Then
move slowly for 45 seconds. Because your work/rest
cycle is relatively short, you can repeat the cycle 10
to 20 times within a single 20-minute workout.

Program 2: Week One: Move for 15 minutes at a pace just below huffing and puffing. Week Two: Move for 20 minutes alternating 1-minute intervals of moving fast and 1-minute intervals of moving slow.

But don't try intervals every time you move. In fact, it's better to train according to how you feel. If you put on your shoes and feel energized, do intervals. If you don't feel like working out, put on your shoes anyway and do a slow, steady burn. Moving slowly is a lot better than not moving at all.

Keeping your activity easy is your number one priority. A gradual progression of beginning slowly and progressing gradually will help you to accomplish that. The next priority is to keep your activity exciting. The best way to beat boredom is variety. Have a selection of workouts to choose from to keep you and your body from burning out.

Ab-Isolation Training

Your ab-isolation training may be performed at home, in your office, or in the gym. Train your abs no more than every other day. Your ab-isolation exercises should take no longer than a few minutes.

How hard you train your abs is more important than how long. Go for "the burn" occasionally, but if your stomach muscles feel uncomfortable for a couple of days, you went too far.

Your Personal Trainer

Start each movement slowly, as if you are in slow motion.

If you find yourself in a seated position and you only have a few minutes to train your abs, try this quick, 15-second ab-toning circuit. Circuit training is when you move from one exercise to the next as quickly as possible. Hold each position for 3 seconds.

Chair Circuit

Lean back until your stomach muscles contract, but don't touch the back of your chair. Then, without rest, bring your right foot off of the floor and your right knee toward your chest. Do the same with your left leg. For the final exercise, press your right forearm into your right armrest. Do the same with your left forearm.

In 15 seconds you worked all of your ab muscles. If you have more time, simply do another circuit of the same routine. Three sets would be perfect.

Perform 3 ab-isolation exercises 3 times a week. Target each muscle with a specific exercise. Do 3 exercises per workout—one for your front abs, one for your side abs, and one that targets all of your stomach muscles simultaneously. Mix and match. Your abs love to be challenged from different angles and intensities. Use perfect form to maximize your progress and minimize soreness.

If you are extremely short on time, but you are at home or in the gym, put our ab-isolation exercises together into a floor circuit workout. This method of training keeps your heart rate up so that you tone your abs and lose belly fat simultaneously.

Floor Circuit

Lie on your back and do a set of 10 perfect crunches. Then, without any rest, do a set of 10 reverse crunches. Turn over on your stomach and hold a plank for 10 seconds. By now you might need a breather, so take a 30-second break and a sip of water. Then lie down on your side and hold a side plank for 10 seconds. Switch to your other side and hold a plank for 10 seconds.

And there you have it—a great ab-toning workout in less than 2 minutes (and that included your 30-second break).

Each Week Add Two Reps to Your Program

When you first begin training your abs, they respond to almost any exercise you do. But if you don't continue to challenge them, they stay the same. That is why you should add 2 repetitions per week to your ab-isolation program. Look for visible results in a few weeks.

Get It Right

Don't get caught up with thinking you must have a sensational workout every time you hit the pavement. Everyone has off days.

Add One New Isolation Exercise Each Month

Just as you get bored doing the same things over and over, your abs do, too. When you don't add anything new to your ab-isolation program don't expect to see improvement. Adding one new ab-isolation exercise each month will ignite your progress.

Eating Program

Anybody can go on an exercise program, but changing your eating habits is the key to seeing those abs. To lose the fat that covers your abs, it is more about planning than willpower.

Eat 250 calories less each day than normal.

Most people overeat. Even if you eat healthy foods, you can still eat too much. Your body stores extra fuel as energy in your muscles, energy in your liver, or fat around your stomach. Pay attention to serving and portion sizes.

Eat nutrient-dense foods, not calorically dense.

Eating foods that fuel your ab muscles goes a long way to reducing your waistline. Lean protein is necessary for the growth and repair of your brand new ab muscles.

Below are some sample foods for your eating program. There are hundreds more to choose from.

Sample Foods on the Eating Program

	Lean Protein	Complex Carbs	Fruit
❏	Fish	Corn family	Apricots
❏	Venison	Salad family	Bananas
❏	Turkey	Cruciferous veggies	Strawberries

Water is the ultimate nutrient. Approximately 70 percent of the body is water. Your abdominal muscles are three fourths water.

Drink about 1 milliliter of water per calorie that you burn. That means if you burn 2,000 calories working out, you need to drink an additional 2 liters of water.

If you want to shed fat around your abs, pay attention to what you eat and when you eat. Replacing both fluids and energy are important if you are trying to recover and prepare for tomorrow's ab workout.

Common thought used to be that if you ate fat, you wore it. And Americans eat plenty of fat; especially omega-six fatty acids. Avoid trans fat, limit saturated fat, and add omega-three fatty acids to your diet. Now we know that eating omega-three fatty acids actually helps you to trim those abs. Omega-three fatty acids are the good fats. You can find them in nuts, fish, flaxseed, and canola oil.

You were not meant to sit around for long periods. Find ways to get moving. Read for a while and then go for a walk. Take a stretch break or do some calisthenics. Once you begin to move, without fail your diet magically improves. Your body and brain get in synch and you make better food choices. You feel better, look refreshed, and your muscles get toned and tight. You feel like an athlete and fuel your muscles with the nutrients they need. The snowball continues until your abs finally look the way you want them to. And once you're there, maintaining those sleek, sexy abs is easy.

Reading, Viewing, Surfing

Abs are here to stay. People never get tired of searching for new ways to get sleek, sexy abs. Look through any fitness magazine or exercise DVD or search health-related websites and you will find something about abdominals or ab-training.

If you're fanatical about achieving a flat, toned stomach, do your research and check out the magazines, DVDs, videos, and websites below.

Magazines to Motivate Your Ab Training

Looking at photos of magazine models with amazing abs may inspire you to get your ab workout in. You may notice that there is nothing new with regard to ab training, but at least you can try some tips if they are substantiated by research.

Muscle and Fitness Hers

Yoga Journal

Weight Watchers

Men's Health

Women's Health

Oxygen Fitness magazine

Videos to Change Up Your Abs Routine

There are only so many ways to train your abs. But these videos are particularly informative about training your back as well.

Leslie Sansone's Short Cuts Abs

The Firm: 5-Day Abs

Gilad's Quick Fit Abs

Karen Voight's Core Essentials

Best Abs on Earth

Websites to Bolster Your Workout

Check out some of these sites to get your eating program on track and to fine-tune your ab training.

Berkeley Wellness Letter
www.berkeleywellness.com

American Council on Exercise
www.acefitness.org

Nutrition Data
www.nutritiondata.com

Fitness World
www.fitnessworld.com

Tom Seabourne's Website
www.tomseabourne.com

Index

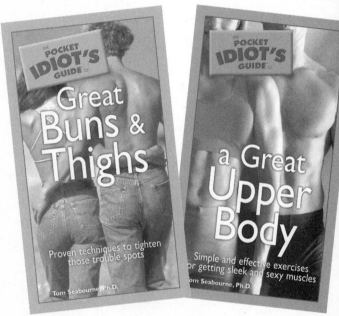